"Rarely has a book been needed as urgen[...]
been better qualified to write it. I urge all [...]
be able to provide a truly biblical respons[...]
of our day."

—**Tim Challies,** author of *Seasons of Sorrow:*
The Pain of Loss and the Comfort of God

"A penetrating analysis of so-called 'medical aid in dying,' a rapidly expanding practice that promises salvation from suffering but expresses despair. Read this remarkable book to remember, and help others to remember, why Christians can face suffering and death with patience and hope."

—**Farr Curlin, MD,** Josiah C. Trent Professor of Medical Humanities,
Trent Center for Bioethics, Humanities, and History of Medicine;
codirector, Theology, Medicine and Culture Initiative, Duke Divinity School

"This is the kind of contribution to the debate that we need a great deal more of: a practicing physician who, having learned of life and death from his patients and his practice, has made use of widely read reflection to interpret them. The inherent contradictions of a practice based on despair appear with a clarity that perhaps no philosopher or theologian could give them."

—**Oliver O'Donovan,** professor emeritus of Christian ethics and
practical theology, University of Edinburgh

"Possibly the most important ethical issue of our time, the practice of offering assisted dying makes an implicit claim about how we regard the value of human life. *How Should We then Die?* will help laity to understand the legal, medical, ethical, and theological matters at stake in the debate."

—**Kathryn Greene-McCreight,** priest affiliate of Christ Church,
New Haven; author of *Darkness Is My Only Companion:*
A Christian Response to Mental Illness

"According to advocates, physician-assisted death acknowledges and protects the dignity of sufferers. With clarity, conciseness, and compassion, Dr. Ewan Goligher demonstrates how the secular narrative upon which the practice rests actually devalues humans and robs us of meaning and well-grounded hope. I hope this impressive work of moral reasoning and Christian witness will be read and pondered by medical professionals, patients, and those who love them."

—**Keith W. Plummer,** dean, School of Divinity, Cairn University

"Through clear, measured, and probing reflections, Dr. Goligher offers a diagnostic guide that helps us understand why euthanasia is deceptively attractive to those who are suffering or fear the loss of what they consider a life worth living. Combining Christian faith and reason, analysis and experience, his insights shine needed light on how we should think about death, dignity, and the value of every human life and how euthanasia medicalizes death and devalues life. His wise counsel reaffirms the need for faith, hope, and love to address our darkest fears and satisfy our deepest yearnings for comfort, both in life and in death."

—**Lauris C. Kaldjian, MD,** director, Program in Bioethics and Humanities, Richard M. Caplan Chair in Biomedical Ethics and Medical Humanities, and professor, Department of Internal Medicine, Carver College of Medicine, University of Iowa

"Do all humans have intrinsic value, or can humans who have diminished capacities be rightly killed by doctors? Is death the final end, or are there reasons to suppose that human intelligence and freedom entail the possession of a spiritual soul and a God-given vocation in all stages of life? This clear and brilliant book answers these questions (and much more) from the perspectives of reason and faith, powerfully combatting the despair that makes us so terribly vulnerable to the false logic of 'mercy' killing."

—**Matthew Levering,** James N. Jr. and Mary D. Perry Chair of Theology, Mundelein Seminary

"It is tragic that my country, Canada, has become a world leader in offering death as a 'treatment.' What began as a last option for adults hobbled by incurable disease and intractable pain with death foreseeable has become, in seven short years, a possible response to chronic disease and mental illnesses with the boundaries extended to 'mature minors.' And still there is no bottom to the descent in sight. A recent poll suggests that almost two-thirds of Canadians supported physician-assisted death as a remedy for homelessness! People, and especially physicians, with the courage to stand athwart the mob and say, 'NO!' are in short supply. I am grateful for Dr. Ewan Goligher's brief, accessible guide for Christians (and others) who greet this brave new world with grave misgivings. Buy this book for yourself, your friends, your church."

—**Tim Perry,** professor of theology and church ministries, Providence Theological Seminary, Otterburne, Canada

HOW SHOULD WE THEN DIE?

A Christian Response to
Physician-Assisted Death

HOW SHOULD WE THEN DIE?

A Christian Response to Physician-Assisted Death

EWAN C. GOLIGHER

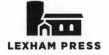

LEXHAM PRESS

*How Should We Then Die?: A Christian Response
to Physician-Assisted Death*

Copyright 2024 Ewan C. Goligher

Lexham Press, 1313 Commercial St., Bellingham, WA 98225
LexhamPress.com

Print ISBN 9781683597476
Digital ISBN 9781683597483
Library of Congress Control Number 2023944724

Lexham Editorial: Todd Hains, Katrina Smith
Cover Design: Jonathan Myers
Typesetting: Abigail Stocker

For my beloved wife, Rachel

Who embodies to me faith, hope, and love
'Til death do us part
(And then only for a moment)

CONTENTS

PRAYER FOR
THE NUMBER OF OUR DAYS

In the name of the Father and of the Son
and of the Holy Spirit.
Amen.

Lord, you have been our dwelling place
    in all generations.
Before the mountains were brought forth,
    or ever you had formed the earth and the world,
    from everlasting to everlasting you are God.
You return man to dust
    and say, "Return, O children of man!"
For a thousand years in your sight
    are but as yesterday when it is past,
    or as a watch in the night.
You sweep them away as with a flood;
    they are like a dream,
    like grass that is renewed in the morning:
in the morning it flourishes and is renewed;
    in the evening it fades and withers.

For we are brought to an end by your anger;
    by your wrath we are dismayed.
You have set our iniquities before you,
    our secret sins in the light of your presence.
For all our days pass away under your wrath;
    we bring our years to an end like a sigh.
The years of our life are seventy,
    or even by reason of strength eighty;
yet their span is but toil and trouble;
    they are soon gone, and we fly away.
Who considers the power of your anger,
    and your wrath according to the fear of you?
So teach us to number our days
    that we may get a heart of wisdom.
Return, O Lord! How long?
    Have pity on your servants!
Satisfy us in the morning with your steadfast love,
    that we may rejoice and be glad all our days.
Make us glad for as many days
    as you have afflicted us,
    and for as many years as we have seen evil.
Let your work be shown to your servants,
    and your glorious power to their children.
Let the favor of the Lord our God be upon us,
    and establish the work of our hands upon us;
    yes, establish the work of our hands!

Psalm 90

Glory be to the Father and to the Son
    and to the Holy Spirit;
As it was in the beginning, is now,
    and will be forever. Amen.

Almighty God and Father,
our lives are like the flowers which flourish in the field;
when the wind blows over them, they are gone,
and that place remembers them no more.
In life, so teach us to number our days
that we might gain a heart of wisdom;
in death, hold us fast in your love
that we might not be forgotten;
and at the last bring us to share fully in the resurrection.
These things we ask in the name
of him who died and rose again,
that he might be the Lord of the dead and the living,
Jesus Christ,
who lives and reigns with you and the Holy Spirit,
one God,
now and forever.
Amen.[1]

I

WHY NOT?

A ROUND THE TIME that the legalization of euthanasia became a matter of public discussion in Canada, I was having lunch with a summer research student who was working with me. In the course of our conversation, we started chatting about physician-assisted death. He was a future medical student and would soon be deciding his own view on the matter, and I was curious to understand what he thought about it.

It wasn't difficult for him to decide the question.

"Why not?" he said. "If that's what they want, why not?"

I was a bit taken aback, that it should seem so easy to answer, so obvious that it would be OK for doctors to end a patient's life. But the way in which the matter was decided for him spoke volumes about the way our society decides what is right or wrong. So long as something feels right to us, so long as it is desirable to us, then there is no reason to think it is wrong, even when it comes to ending a life.

I also realized it was not so easy for me to answer his question, "Why not?" If the value of our existence depends entirely on whether we want to exist, and if our natural right to life can simply be waived if we don't want to be alive, then what basis could we have to say that physician-assisted death is wrong? For our diverse, multicultural, and pluralistic society, where right and wrong and good and evil are matters of personal preference ("you do you"), it is awfully hard to come up with a good reason against causing death if that is what the patient wants. To answer "Why not?" concerning physician-assisted death is to take up much deeper issues about what makes us matter, how we decide what is right and wrong, and why we are alive at all. We can't really talk about death without talking about life.

This book is an attempt to offer an answer to the question "Why not?"

A Moral Question We All Must Face

Should doctors help patients end their own life? Is it right and good to cause death (to kill) out of mercy for suffering? Over the last decades, Western society has seen a marked rise in interest and support for the idea that doctors should be allowed (even expected) to facilitate suicide or cause death for their patients under certain conditions. This shift in social values, together with an aging population, means that all of us, whether or not we work in health care, will be forced to face this question. Every one of us will eventually face illness, suffering, and death at some point, and we will have to decide whether we would consider seeking and obtaining assistance from a doctor to end our life.

This short book is written specifically to help Christians think about this question. Why write specifically for Christians? In the first place, those who follow Jesus are called to be deeply committed to doing and being good. We aim to live a life of love for God and for neighbor. In following Jesus, we are to make others' interests our own. As Christians, compassion toward suffering is one of our most deeply held values, and we look to Jesus's life and ministry as the model of compassion and mercy. We are therefore deeply concerned to address and relieve suffering where possible, and we are naturally inclined to support any means of doing so. Christianity has traditionally opposed physician-assisted death, but its proponents advocate for it as a matter of compassion and mercy and of respect for those who are suffering. The question of whether causing death out of mercy represents an appropriate and compassionate means of relieving suffering is therefore of urgent interest to us.

Second, Christians share a particular understanding of the value of humanity. The Christian cosmic metanarrative of creation, fall, redemption, and glory—sometimes referred to simply as "the gospel"—gives us a particular understanding of who we are, where we've come from, what we are for, and why and how much we matter. As we will see, this shared understanding of ourselves becomes profoundly relevant to the question of causing death out of mercy. Christians must therefore be concerned to understand how the truth about humanity revealed in the gospel of Christ applies to the question of assisted death.

Some may question whether, in a matter of public concern such as medical ethics, it is appropriate to allow one particular personal religious viewpoint to shape one's ethics. Should Christians allow their Christian beliefs to inform their views on medical ethics in a society where church and state are supposed to be separate? This is a particularly important question for Christian doctors and nurses, who by virtue of their professional responsibilities toward patients operate in the public square. Our views on the ethics of assisted death affects not only ourselves but also our patients. Given that our patients often do not share our faith in Christ, can we allow Christian commitment to shape how we care for them? Many would say that deriving one's professional ethics from Christian belief (or other personal religious convictions) inappropriately imposes the strictures of religion on the patient. Such an imposition seems especially egregious given the vulnerability of the patient and the power dynamics of the doctor-patient relationship. Christians, therefore, seem to face a conflict between personal religious conviction and professional ethical obligations.

In this book, I will address this apparent conflict in two ways. First, I will present arguments that proceed from basic moral starting points that nearly everyone accepts and shares, irrespective of their particular religious (or nonreligious) outlook. Having made such a general moral argument, I will proceed to show how Christian belief grounds, strengthens, and enriches one's understanding of the issues addressed in the argument.

Second, I will argue that everyone is conflicted, including health-care professionals who don't hold to any traditional religious beliefs. I will explore the ways in which our view on the ethics of assisted death is unavoidably shaped by our understanding of who we are, where we come from, and what happens after we die. The issue of physician-assisted death actually serves as a case study to highlight the ways in which a secular belief system (traditionally regarded as nonreligious because it functions without reference to God or concern for the afterlife) is really just another religious viewpoint. "Religion" is a much broader concept than many realize; even nonbelievers have beliefs about human value, the meaning of life (or its lack thereof), and what happens after we die. When it comes to the ethics of death and dying, the influence of one's personal religion is pretty much unavoidable.

II

WHY ASSISTED DEATH?

T HE MEMORY OF her agony is etched indelibly in my mind. When I met her, she was doubled over in pain, kneeling at the side of the bed as if pleading with God for mercy. Her cancer had invaded the bottom of her spine, rendering the bone fragile and unstable. The bottom of the spine had collapsed inward, crushing the delicate nerves at the base of the spinal cord. And so she was in agony, finding only minimal relief by kneeling and doubling over. She had been in that position for days, unable to sleep and without relief, and had now come to the hospital for help. With tears of exhaustion and desperation, she pleaded for relief.

That night I struggled to manage her pain, trying different drugs and doses. Finally, with a continuous infusion of hydromorphone (a morphine-like drug), I was able to achieve some control of the pain. I remember going to check on her in the middle of the night. She was finally lying on her side, comfortably asleep. I slowly exhaled a sigh of relief. I was only a young resident at the time, and her pain had made a powerful impression on me. Indeed, I have rarely seen such a severe pain crisis any time since. Pain robbed that woman of her dignity; it left her desperate and broken in spirit. So long as she was in agony, she could think of nothing but freedom from the pain. The relief of her pain restored her dignity, allowed her to breathe, to rest, to be human.

The Indignity of Suffering

It is sometimes said that we fear dying as much, or even more, than we fear death itself. The possibility of enduring raw physical agony on the journey toward death fills us with real apprehension. In truth, medicine has powerful tools at its disposal to relieve or control physical suffering, and modern palliative medicine is entirely devoted to maximizing comfort and dignity for patients as they journey toward death, holistically addressing physical, emotional, and spiritual needs. But many people are still largely unaware of the possibilities of effective pain and symptom control for the dying, and it is a sad travesty that training and resources are still not sufficient to ensure universal access to high-quality palliative care even in some developed countries. Hence, in our imagination, the journey toward death retains the specter of uncontrolled suffering, and the possibility of a "death with dignity" by having your doctor cause your death in the manner and timing of your choosing seems like an appropriate means of avoiding needless suffering. We don't want pain, suffering, and dying to rob us of our dignity.

Dignity is a big concept; it concerns our sense of our own value, the value that others perceive in us, and how we should be treated in accordance with that value. Of course, you do not need to have your life ended by your doctor or to commit suicide in order to die with dignity. But the essential argument for physician-assisted death is that the option of physician-assisted death gives patients the confidence that they can avoid suffering and thereby maintain their dignity up until their very last moments. By offering to cause the patient's death upon their request, we allow patients to take control over the manner and timing of their death, so that they need not live in fear of suffering during the dying process.

Defining Physician-Assisted Death

Clear definitions are essential. By physician-assisted death, I am referring to intentional and deliberate actions on the part of the physician aimed at causing the death of the patient. These are actions where death is the stated purpose and goal of the intervention. Two different kinds of actions by physicians to cause death may be distinguished. Physicians may provide a prescription for a lethal dose of a drug that the patient then administers to herself. The physician makes the lethal drug available, but the patient must take it by her own hand. This is traditionally referred to as physician-assisted suicide. Alternately, the physician may directly administer the lethal dose to the patient, usually intravenously. This is traditionally referred to as euthanasia. From an ethical standpoint, there is no real distinction between physician-assisted suicide and euthanasia, since in both cases the doctor is deliberately and knowingly acting to cause the patient's death and is responsible for the patient's death. There is, however, an important practical distinction between these two kinds of physician-assisted death; patients seem reluctant to self-administer a lethal drug and to actually cause their own death. In jurisdictions where both physician-assisted suicide and euthanasia are legal, patients overwhelmingly opt for the latter; they seem to greatly prefer having the doctor administer the lethal drug. In this way, prohibiting euthanasia while legalizing physician-assisted suicide creates a practical limitation to widespread adoption of physician-assisted death—many patients find it difficult to bring themselves to cause their own death.

Physician-assisted suicide and euthanasia can be clearly distinguished from other issues in end-of-life care or decision-making such as palliative care, terminal sedation, or withholding or withdrawing life-sustaining therapies. None of these practices necessarily require the doctor to deliberately aim at causing the patient's death. Death may follow the decision to withdraw life support (which is not really an action but rather the cessation of action), but the actual cause of death is the underlying illness. Life-sustaining treatments are not discontinued in order to bring about the patient's death; rather, they are discontinued because it is recognized that they are no longer effective or appropriate. As an intensive care specialist, I have been involved in this decision many times. In these cases, patients are persistently critically ill despite aggressive life-sustaining therapies, and it becomes clear that the patient will not recover. I can assure you that I have never withdrawn life support specifically in order to cause a patient's death. Of course, were I to withdraw life support in order to cause the patient's death, then my action would be the ethical equivalent of euthanasia. The intention, or goal, of the action is the key distinguishing feature.

The act of deliberately causing the death of another person has traditionally been referred to as homicide, and the act of deliberately causing one's own death is traditionally called suicide. Advocates for physician-assisted death dislike and avoid these terms because they are heavily freighted with negative value judgments or stigma—"medical homicide" doesn't sound good, even if it is the most accurate term to describe what happens with euthanasia. Advocates argue that because a health-care professional is administering death according to the patient's voluntary request, the act is something much closer to suicide than homicide. But the word "suicide" is also avoided because, again, it makes us uncomfortable. Advocates for physician-assisted death argue that it is different from suicide because it feels different from committing suicide. The American Association of Suicidology contends that suicide and physician-assisted death are categorically different because they generally involve very different experiences of dying.[2] Suicide is committed alone, through violent means, in isolation from others, and feels like "self-destruction" (their term). On the other hand, they suggest that physician-assisted death feels like an act of "self-preservation" (their term) that aims at preserving the person's sense of dignity, is performed in comfort by a trained professional, and is often enacted in the company of supportive family and friends.

There is no doubt that the experience of physician-assisted death is probably quite different from the tragic loneliness of acting alone to cause one's own death by other (possibly more violent) means. And, for an organization such as the American Association of Suicidology, it is important to distinguish between physician-assisted death and suicide because they do not want the legalization of physician-assisted death to undermine their efforts at suicide prevention.

Yet mere differences in the typical experience of death between physician-assisted death and suicide do not resolve the basic moral question of whether it is appropriate to deliberately cause someone's death. Is it right and good to end an innocent person's life upon their request so long as one is doing so in the most humane manner possible? Put simply, is physician-assisted death a morally appropriate and praiseworthy type of suicide or homicide? Is homicide appropriate (praiseworthy, even) when it is performed by a doctor at the patient's invitation and with the good intention of relieving suffering? Why not? This is the question we must answer.

Why Some People Want Physician-Assisted Death

Before we examine the "why not" of physician-assisted death we should seek to understand the "why." We naturally find life precious. To seek death seems difficult and foreign to us. Why, then, do patients want to have their life ended by their doctor? Because physician-assisted death has been legal in several locations around the world for some time, we can look back and understand why patients in those places are seeking euthanasia. A number of key studies have been published, looking at this question. Patients who were seeking and preparing to obtain euthanasia were asked why they wanted to have their life ended. These studies provide invaluable insights for us as we seek to understand physician-assisted death.

In these studies,[3] most patients (more than 90 percent) who seek assisted death say that the main reason for ending their life is a loss of autonomy, the sense that they are no longer able to control their lives or circumstances. Most (more than 80 percent) also cited an inability to engage in enjoyable activities and a sense of loss of personal dignity. Some express concern about being a burden on family, friends, or caregivers. Only a minority (less than 30 percent) of patients sought assisted death because of "inadequate pain control or concern about it" (and it is likely that only a small number of those patients truly had inadequate pain control).

A study from a Canadian hospital published shortly after the legalization of physician-assisted death in Canada reports,

> Those who received [medical aid in dying] tended to be white and relatively affluent and indicated that loss of autonomy was the primary reason for their request.

Other common reasons included the wish to avoid
burdening others or losing dignity and the intolera-
bility of not being able to enjoy one's life. Few patients
cited inadequate control of pain or other symptoms.[4]

Studies in Europe have reported similar findings.[5] Across
multiple studies in multiple countries, pain and other symptoms are consistently not the main reason for seeking physician-assisted death. Rather, it seems that patients want to
have their life ended because they no longer find a reason to
live. They aren't in control anymore, they can't do what they
want to do, they feel like a burden, they feel hopeless, and
they find that an intolerable affront to their dignity. There
is simply no point in going on.

Another consistent finding from studies of patients who
seek euthanasia is that they are generally from a specific
group in society—wealthy, white, nonreligious people.[6]
Advocates sometimes cite this observation in support of
physician-assisted death because it is taken to mean that
these patients are not from so-called vulnerable or marginalized populations. They are not being taken advantage of
or forced to obtain physician-assisted death. A colleague
who has been involved in providing physician-assisted
death reassures me that these patients are "captains of
industry," people who are used to being independent and
in control. They are not vulnerable to coercion. Nobody is
making them choose assisted death.

But is it possible that we might fail to understand the true nature of vulnerability? What if vulnerability to physician-assisted death arises from within ourselves, rather than from external social forces? What if vulnerability to assisted death has more to do with having an outlook on life that makes it difficult to find a point in living with suffering? What if, after a lifetime of being in control, we cannot tolerate losing control? What if we lack the resources offered by religious or spiritual beliefs and community to make sense out of suffering and to transcend it? What if our vulnerability is not social but rather psychological and spiritual? That a very specific group of people are predisposed to seek physician-assisted death, a group that is comparatively less vulnerable to economic and social pressures and also comparatively less religious, raises the distinct possibility that existential, philosophical, and spiritual concerns—problems of meaning and significance in the face of suffering and loss—are the real sources of vulnerability to the desire for death.

The Death of Gillian Bennett

One of the most poignant suicide notes I have read was written by Gillian Bennett. A brilliant and articulate woman, a trained psychotherapist, she was diagnosed with dementia and began to experience the resulting limitations, weakness, and frailty. She decided to end her own life in order to avoid experiencing further decline. She wrote about her decision on a webpage, deadatnoon.com, prior to the legalization of assisted death in Canada. The story of her death and her reasons for choosing death were widely discussed in the media. Her words help us to understand the point of view of a patient seeking physician-assisted death.

> I will take my life today around noon. It is time. Dementia is taking its toll and I have nearly lost myself. I have nearly lost me. ... I have known that I have dementia, a progressive loss of memory and judgment, for three years. It is a stealthy, stubborn and oh-so reliable disease. ... Ever so gradually at first, much faster now, I am turning into a vegetable. I find it hard to keep in my mind that my granddaughter is coming in three day's time and not today. "Where do we keep the X?" (coffee / milkshake-maker / backspace on my keyboard / the book I was just reading) happens all the time. I have constantly to monitor what I say in an attempt not to make some gross error of judgment.
>
> There comes a time, in the progress of dementia, when one is no longer competent to guide one's own affairs. I want out before the day when I can no longer assess my situation, or take action to bring my life to an end. There could also come a time when I simply must make a decision based on my deteriorating physical health. I do not like hospitals—they are dirty places. Any doctor will tell you to stay out of them if you possibly can. I would not want a fall, a stroke, or some

unforeseen complication to mess up my decision to cost Canada as little as possible in my declining years.

Understand that I am giving up nothing that I want by committing suicide. All I lose is an indefinite number of years of being a vegetable in a hospital setting, eating up the country's money but having not the faintest idea of who I am.

Each of us is born uniquely and dies uniquely. I think of dying as a final adventure with a predictably abrupt end. I know when it's time to leave and I do not find it scary.[7]

According to the website, Gillian Bennett died at 11 a.m. on August 18, 2014, in the presence of her husband. News of her death, and her poignant declaration of her reasons for ending her life, contributed to the growing public support for physician-assisted death. Within a year of her death, the Supreme Court of Canada struck down the criminal code prohibiting physician-assisted death.

So how do we respond to people like Gillian, who find no reason to go on, who want life to be over, and who want to control the manner and timing of their death? Given this "why," which seems so intuitive and plausible in our present social milieu, is there a reasonable "Why not"? To this question we now turn.

III

ASSISTED DEATH DEVALUES PEOPLE

P EOPLE MATTER. REGARDLESS of your view of physician-assisted death, everyone agrees that people matter. Those who advocate for physician-assisted death care about people. They are deeply troubled about the suffering that people endure and the lack of control and the hopelessness that people may feel as they move toward the end of their lives. Those who oppose assisted death care about people—they worry that vulnerable people could easily be persuaded to end their life when they don't really want to die. They worry that people could be made to feel a burden to others, that they would be abused or mistreated, and that a lack of access to good medical care would move them to give up and simply choose to have their life ended. Both sides of this debate about assisted death care deeply about people. They speak and act the way they do because they are persuaded that people matter.

Everyone knows that people matter; it's one of those fundamental and unavoidably true truths, something we feel and know deeply. It is something we cannot not know. Our social media feeds are full of statements and articles and videos decrying the poor treatment of people and demanding the proper treatment of people. Our newspapers are full of stories about the greatness of people or the suffering of people. These social concerns are motivated by a shared conviction that people matter. We widely recognize that people have rights, rights to fair and equal treatment, and that the law ought to recognize these rights so as to ensure that people get the treatment they deserve. When human rights are violated, when people are systematically mistreated, we are troubled, even outraged. When we hear of stories of bullying in schools or exploitation in the workplace, we are deeply troubled, disappointed, saddened. Why? Because people matter, and we feel that very deeply.

Think also of those whom we know most closely and love most deeply—our parents, our siblings, our close friends, family, or neighbors. The closer we are to someone, the more deeply we recognize their value and the more they matter to us. I use that word "recognize" very deliberately: people do not come to matter more merely because we are closer to them. Rather, it is because we are closer to them that we can see more clearly just how much they matter, how precious and valuable they are. They would matter just as much if we did not know them, but we are fortunate to know them well enough to have a deeper appreciation for their value than others might have.

Because we see how much each person matters, we are deeply grieved when we find that people are not being treated according to their true value. We find it a profound travesty when parents fail to value their children or when grown children fail to love and honor their elderly parents. At a park near my home, there is a small statue of a little boy wearing a Superman costume. Jeffrey Baldwin was just six years old when he died of hunger, neglect, and horrific abuse at the hands of his own grandparents, who kept him merely for the social assistance checks they received on his behalf. He was abused and forsaken by his parents, and then his grandparents apparently kept him locked in a room for years with inadequate food and drink, beat him, and forced to drink from a toilet. This tragedy, this unspeakable evil, seems too grotesque to imagine. We are horrified because we recognize that this little boy was of profound value and ought never to have been treated this way. The tragic evil of this story is that little Jeffrey's value was not recognized and that he was not treated in accordance with his true value. Local community members erected a statue in an effort to give dignity to his memory, a little boy dreaming of being a superhero.

People matter.

The Nature of Human Value

When we say that people matter, just what do we mean exactly? We are saying that they are precious, that they are of immense value. But what kind of value do they have? One can distinguish between two kinds of value: extrinsic value and intrinsic value. Extrinsic value refers to value that derives from what something can do for you, such that you find it valuable and it therefore becomes valuable ("value from outside"). Intrinsic value, by contrast, refers to value that arises from the thing in itself ("value from inside").

To appreciate the difference between extrinsic and intrinsic value, we might consider the example of a bicycle. A bicycle is often something we value a great deal; we enjoy riding it, and it gets us around town much faster than if we were to walk. If we were to sell it, it might sell for hundreds or even thousands of dollars because it happens to be in very good condition, and it works beautifully with new components and a nice paint job. Others would pay for it because they would also find it valuable.

But despite its not-insubstantial value, a bicycle can only have extrinsic value, and we can see this in several ways. First, its value depends on its usefulness. If it stopped working, it would no longer be of any value. If we could fix it, then it would be valuable again, but if it is broken beyond repair, then its value is lost. So its value depends on how well it works. Second, the bicycle is replaceable. We could replace it with a different and even better bike, something newer or even more useful to us. Third, we are under no obligation to value the bike, unless we find it valuable or someone else finds it valuable. Nobody will accuse you of failing to value your bike if you decide to sell it to someone else and replace it with another. Rather, it is valuable only if you find it of value. Its value comes from an outside source (from us, the "valuers"). Hence we say that it has only extrinsic value, value from outside. Fourth, we can put a price on it. The price reflects its value in our eyes and in the eyes of others (the market). That we can put a price on it indicates that its value depends on its usefulness to us and others, and that it can be exchanged (replaced) for something else of value to us (i.e., money). It is not priceless.

Another example of something with only extrinsic value would be a smartphone. Your smartphone might seem like one of the most valuable things you have, but only because it is so incredibly useful. As soon as a better, more capable smartphone comes along, you will be happy to replace your smartphone with the new one (as usually happens every two to three years). If you're fortunate, you might be able to sell your phone for a certain price to somebody else to help pay for the new phone. And nobody would consider you unkind or unloving or disrespectful or immoral if you decided to replace your phone. There's no moral obligation or expectation to value your smartphone. In other words, a smartphone has only extrinsic value, value from outside.

We would all agree that the kind of value that people have is very different from that of a bicycle or a smartphone. First, the extent to which people matter does not depend on their usefulness or their function; their value is unconditional. No matter whether someone is athletic or not, smart or not, artistic or not, popular or not, they are profoundly valuable.

Second, unlike a bike or a smartphone, people are irre-placeable. No one person can be replaced or exchanged for another person. When we lose someone, we cannot ever really replace them with another person; each of us is pro-foundly unique in our value.

Third, unlike a bike or a smartphone, people are priceless. Slavery and human trafficking are recognized as great evils because they involve buying and selling people, valuing them only for their utility to others.

Fourth, people have a kind of value that we are obligated to recognize and respect. Their value does not depend on our regard for their value (i.e., value from the outside); rather, we are expected to show regard for their value because the value is already there in their person (value from the inside). We have no obligation to value our bike or our smartphone unless we find them useful, but we always ought to recognize and respect value in people. Treating people as if they don't matter is a failure on our part, because people matter and are valuable whether we appreciate it or not.

In sum, these features of human value—unconditional, priceless, irreplaceable, obligatory—demonstrate that people have intrinsic value, not merely extrinsic value.

To appreciate the significance of intrinsic value, consider the example of bullying. We would all agree that the unpopular kid at school who is bullied on the playground and who has no friends matters just as much as the most popular kid in school. This kid might not be that "useful" to others—befriending him won't make them more popular or connected; it might even hold them back socially. If you were his friend, you might be tempted to "replace" him with another, perhaps someone more attractive and socially connected. But deep down we know that we shouldn't treat people according to whether they are useful or popular or whether they enhance our own personal social status. We know that we can't simply replace them with another person (we certainly wouldn't want them to think that we had replaced them with a different friend, unless we were really trying to hurt them). We know that we are obligated to recognize value in others and that we should treat them in accordance with that value. We should aim to make them feel what they really are: priceless and irreplaceable. That's what makes bullying in person or online so tragic and wrong; it's a deep failure to treat people in accordance with their true intrinsic value.

We may naturally be tempted to ask, Where could this intrinsic value come from? On what basis do we humans have such intrinsic value? I will offer a foundation for the intrinsic value of humans below, but at this point in our argument, we don't need to resolve this question. Everyone agrees that people matter (even if our actions sometimes fail to reflect that truth), and we don't need to explain where our value comes from in order to recognize that we have that value.

The Moral Significance of Intrinsic Human Value

Why is it so important to recognize that people have intrinsic value? These categories—intrinsic and extrinsic value—help us to understand how we ought to treat one another. If people merely had extrinsic value, then it would be okay for us to use them for our own purposes, irrespective of their own needs, desires, and interests, because this is how they would gain (extrinsic) value. But we all recognize that it is wrong to treat people as if they have only extrinsic value. Slavery is an obvious example of the evil of treating people as if they have only extrinsic value. Slavery values people based entirely on their usefulness to others; it puts a price on people based on what they are willing to pay. Slavery treats people as if they are replaceable; one slave can be replaced by a different slave to perform the same useful function. This is morally abhorrent and wrong. Slavery, sex trafficking, exploitation of migrant workers, other abuses of power—are all wrong because they are ways in which some people use other people for their own ends. These practices treat people as if they only had extrinsic value deriving from their temporary usefulness, rather than intrinsic value that obligates us to treat them with dignity.

If people have intrinsic value, we must never treat people merely as means to some other end. A willingness to disregard the intrinsic value of others quickly leads to acts of unspeakable evil—the neglect and abuse of young Jeffrey Baldwin, the abuses inflicted on patients by medical researchers acting outside the bounds of ethics and consent (e.g., the Tuskegee syphilis project), slavery, sex trafficking, migrant worker exploitation, and so on. All these are striking examples of a failure to recognize and respect the intrinsic value of people. These issues, and so many others, trouble us because people are not treated as if they matter. To show disregard for people's intrinsic and inherent value is a great evil.

Of course, we are sometimes tempted to treat others as if they have extrinsic value rather than intrinsic value in more subtle ways. Anytime we use people for our own pleasure or purposes without being equally concerned for their interests or well-being, any time we take advantage of them or leave them feeling used, we are devaluing them because we are treating them as if their value were conditional and dependent and as if they were replaceable. Perhaps we choose to be friends with someone because it will make us more well-connected, or just so they can help us get ahead. We know these things are wrong because we are not treating people in accordance with their true intrinsic value. They may be deeply hurt if they learned that we were using them for our own advantage. We have an obligation to treat people with the respect that accords with their true value.

So when we say that people matter, we are saying that they have intrinsic value, value that is unconditional and independent of circumstance, value that is always there regardless of whether others place any value on them. We are saying that people are priceless and irreplaceable. Therefore, we recognize that we have an obligation to treat people in a certain respectful and dignified way that reflects the fact that they matter. Our actions toward them must correspond to their intrinsic value, and should communicate to them that they are valuable and valued. We affirm this appreciation for their value by showing concern for their interests, needs, values, and goals. We make their interests and concerns our own. In a word, we *love* them in word and in deed to the extent possible to us under the circumstances of our relationship to them. "Love" in this sense does not refer to passive feelings of attraction or desire that we experience; it is a verb that signifies value in action.

If we have intrinsic value, then we are also obligated to value ourselves. All of us are sometimes tempted to forget our intrinsic value and to regard ourselves as if we only have extrinsic value. We are sometimes tempted to think that the value of our existence depends on our usefulness to ourselves or to others. If we no longer feel useful in life or if we begin to feel that we are a burden to others, we start to doubt our value and to feel worthless. But if we have intrinsic value, then we are obligated to value ourselves. We must recognize our own unconditional, intrinsic value. The tragedy of the human condition is that we may be inclined to doubt our own value. Our perception of our own value may be distorted, and we may base our sense of our own value entirely on how others treat us or how well we are able to perform for others. The love that others show to us helps us to remember and to see more clearly our own value. When others show us by their actions that we are priceless and irreplaceable, it helps us to see our true value more clearly. Reminding others of their intrinsic value is the essence of loving our neighbor.

The Value of Persons and the Value of Life

The next step in our argument is to appreciate the inseparable connection between the value of a person and the value of their existence. To say that something is of value is to say that it is good that it exists. If something is valuable, it is better that it exists than if it did not exist. You cannot assert that something is valuable while also asserting that it would be better for it not to exist. That would be a logical contradiction, an absurdity. On the other hand, if we say that it doesn't matter whether something exists, then we are also saying that it is not of any real value. Imagine the affront you would feel if someone told you that they didn't care whether you existed. That would of course lead you to believe that they did not value you very much at all.

So there is a deep and inseparable connection between our regard for something's value and our regard for its existence. Having value entails that existence is good. The corollary is that if we are unconcerned about its existence, then we do not value it. If we act to render something nonexistent, we are necessarily demonstrating that we do not regard the thing in itself as having value; otherwise, we would not destroy it. And if we value something, we will be concerned for it to continue to exist.

Of course, things that have only extrinsic value—bikes, smartphones, and so on—may lose their usefulness and hence their value, and we may cease to be concerned for their existence. As long as we value them, we are very concerned for their existence (we don't want to lose them or have them stolen!). But once they have lost their value to us, we are no longer so concerned for their existence. Indeed, we may prefer to see them recycled rather than keep them. But things that have intrinsic value do not lose their value, and so their existence never ceases to be good or important. Accordingly, we are obligated always to have regard for the existence of things that have intrinsic value.

Imagine, for example, that you are the curator of the Louvre Museum in Paris. A famously wealthy but eccentric art collector approaches you with an offer to purchase Leonardo da Vinci's famous painting, the *Mona Lisa*, for vast sums of money. Inquiring what he plans to do with the painting, you discover that he intends to cut it into smaller pieces and sell off the individual pieces at a profit. Of course, you will instantly refuse the offer of purchase. The *Mona Lisa* is so precious, so valuable, that the possibility of it ceasing to exist is utterly unthinkable. If it were to cease to exist (say, because of a museum fire), it would be regarded by the entire world as an unspeakable tragedy.

The connection between value and existence is especially clear when we are forced to come to terms with the death of those we love. How many times I have sat before the wives, husbands, parents, and children of my critically ill patients to utter those unspeakable words, "I'm afraid he's not going to make it." The pain etched on their faces, the tears, the weeping, the broken sobs, the numbed silence, the unendurable grief—all speak to the depth of loss that they are experiencing and hence the depth of value of their loved one. Sometimes I see patients die alone, cut off from loved ones or with no one to mourn them. That in itself feels like an even greater tragedy. When something of such value passes out of existence, there ought to be mourning.

So when we say that people matter, we are also saying that it is good that they exist. If people have intrinsic value, then it is always good that they exist. And if we insist that they really matter—that they have deep, intrinsic, inherent value—then the cessation of their existence (their death) must always be regarded as a terrible tragedy.

The value of a human person and the value of her life are inseparably connected. To speak or to act as if it would be better for a person not to exist is to declare that they have lost their value and to deny that they have intrinsic value.

Assisted Death Denies
Intrinsic Human Value

It is perhaps not difficult to see now how these arguments bear on the question of whether assisted death is right and good.

Proponents of assisted death argue that bringing about the patient's death is a way of showing respect for those who are suffering, a method of upholding their dignity and value in the face of the difficulties and indignities that disability, illness, or dying impose on us. Assisted death purports to uphold the value of persons by empowering them to choose when and how they should die. The question, then, is whether the act of deliberately causing death truly accords with intrinsic human value. Can you say that people really matter when you cause them not to exist?

Of course, assisted death is not the same as murder in that the person has requested that their life be ended. The person performing assisted death (whom I will refer to as the operator) is not imposing her will on the patient or violating her autonomy. The patient herself has decided that it would be better for her not to exist. And in administering the lethal agent, the operator tacitly assents to this decision and expresses a concrete endorsement of the patient's decision. For this reason, assisted death is said to be "patient-centered," for it gives the patient what they want, even if that is a desire for nonexistence.

In providing or administering the lethal agent, the operator inevitably expresses a belief about whether it is good for the person to exist. By intentionally causing the death of the person who has requested death from them, they show that they believe that it is good for that person not to exist. After all, we are supposed to call assisted death the right thing to do in such cases. We would not perform assisted death unless we thought that, all things considered, it was better for the patient to be dead than alive. The assisted-suicide regime in every jurisdiction where it is legal engages a complex set of criteria as to who is eligible—that is, those for whom death would be a good and appropriate thing. In Canada, you are deemed eligible for assisted suicide if your suffering is unbearable to you and death is either reasonably foreseeable or you have a physical disability (these criteria may soon expand to include those with mental illness). According to the law, I am not eligible for assisted suicide, but I personally know others who would be eligible. The law holds that death is not good for me but might possibly be good for them. Eligibility for assisted suicide implies the possible goodness of nonexistence; it at least implies that one's continued existence is not necessarily good.

What, then, does this say about the value of those who receive assisted death or who are potentially eligible for assisted death in comparison to those who are not eligible? Those for whom existence is deemed optional cannot possibly have the same value as those for whom existence is deemed essential. And if the existence of some persons is regarded as optional, then they do not have unconditional intrinsic value. Indeed, since existence could become optional for any of us (if we were to develop a serious disability or chronic illness, then we would become potentially eligible for assisted death), this would imply that nobody really has unconditional intrinsic value. As we have seen, if something has intrinsic, inherent, and unconditional value, then it is always good that it exists. If it is not always good that it exists, then it cannot have intrinsic, inherent, and unconditional value. Instead, if we have any value at all, that value would have to be extrinsic and conditional and dependent on some "valuer."

So an endorsement of assisted death necessarily implies support for the view that people have extrinsic value but not intrinsic value. People matter, but they don't really, absolutely matter. We have some value, but not the sort of fundamental, intrinsic value that we might initially have believed we had. In seeking to have our own existence ended, we are not regarding ourselves as irreplaceable and priceless treasures, the loss of which is an unspeakable tragedy. In offering assisted death, the operator necessarily endorses and supports this (de)valuation.

Another way of seeing how assisted death undermines the value of people is by recognizing that it treats people as a means to an end (in other words, it uses people for some other purpose). It achieves its purpose—the elimination of suffering—by destroying the sufferer. Indeed, it cannot achieve its end apart from this means. So the sufferer is treated as a means, not an end in himself. The sufferer is used to achieve some other goal. That goal might be one that the sufferer has endorsed or preferred, but that does not alter the fact that the sufferer is used for that purpose.

We are forced to conclude that assisted death is not compatible with human value in the deep sense—value that is intrinsic, inherent, and unconditional. Support for assisted death requires that we adopt a lesser view of human value. If causing people to cease to exist is good and right, then the value of our persons is at bottom merely extrinsic and conditional. Assisted death devalues people.

Autonomy and Intrinsic Human Value

Now, proponents of assisted suicide purport to care very much about human value. Their support for assisted death, they insist, is motivated by the value of those who suffer. They try to reconcile assisted suicide with human value by insisting that assisting suicide is a matter of respect for autonomy. The value of the person seeking and receiving assisted suicide might be contingent and dependent on a valuer but that valuer is the person themselves. Respect is shown by treating the person as the basis of their own value. By regarding the person as the source of their own value, the person appears to be accorded deep significance and importance. By recognizing them as having the authority to determine their own value (empowering their autonomy), we appear to accord them profound importance and value.

But this kind of value is a deception, for it still denies that we have real intrinsic, inherent value. By making our personal value depend on our own preferences and self-regard, we might appear to have intrinsic value. After all, isn't this "value from inside"? In actual fact, it is extrinsic value, because the value is dependent and conditional on our self-regard. When we treat ourselves as the foundation of our own value, we are forcing ourselves to bear an unbearable weight. If we find ourselves in a situation where we are unable or unwilling to value ourselves, then we lose our value. If we are of no use to ourselves, then we really are useless. If my existence is bad for me, then it really is bad to exist. By contrast, if I had intrinsic value, I would be obligated as valuer to value myself. But if I do not have such intrinsic value, then I am under no obligation to value myself, and I am free to do with myself as I please, no matter how self-destructive my choices might be. But such freedom comes at the cost of acknowledging that we have no intrinsic value.

This loss of intrinsic value and this reliance on our own will to assert our extrinsic value creates huge problems for our self-worth. I might demand respect from others, but what basis do I have to merit respect from myself? My own value is at bottom a matter of sheer choice. Such an arbitrary basis for human value is incredibly thin and cannot withstand any of the pressures that tempt us to devalue ourselves—we have little response to anything that leads us to doubt our self-worth, our significance, or the meaningfulness of our existence. Certainly we cannot look to others for reassurance of our value—what authority do they have to recognize value in us if we do not recognize it in ourselves? If I am the sole basis for determining my value, then I have no real cause to assign myself any value. In making ourselves the source of our own value, we undermine any basis for actually being valuable.

And the risk here is that, knowing this, others begin to doubt or deny our value as well. And if they do so, on what basis can we require them to respect our value? If our value depends on respect for our autonomy, on what does respect for our autonomy depend? After all, our autonomy only matters if we matter in the first place. If we claim that recognition of our value derives from respect for our autonomy, and if respect for our autonomy depends on the recognition of our value, then we find ourselves offering a circular argument that commands no respect at all. Any attempt to ground our value in our autonomy must falter because the obligation to respect personal autonomy presumes our personal value in the first place. We respect autonomy because people matter, not the other way around. Hence, denying intrinsic human value undermines the obligation to respect our autonomy and choices.

In any case, we all know that human value is real. People really do matter. Our value is not contingent or dependent on some arbitrary expression of preference. When we see people in difficult circumstances struggling to value themselves, we wish that they could see how much they actually matter. The young child subjected to neglect and mistreatment at the hands of abusive grandparents may struggle to love and value himself; this we regard as a tragedy, for he truly is valuable, even if he cannot see it. We do not allow people to treat themselves as means to ends by, for example, selling themselves into slavery. People really matter, and therefore our value is not dependent merely on our self-regard. Because our value is intrinsic, it is not a matter of mere choice. Rather, because we are intrinsically valuable we are obligated to value ourselves in accordance with our true value.

Dependence and Value

Human value cannot be rescued by making the individual the grounds for their own value. We are too weak, too frail, too vulnerable to circumstance to be a firm foundation for our own value and significance. And this is a burden we need not bear, for we are intrinsically valuable, no matter how we feel about ourselves. Yet the tragedy of the human condition is that we are prone to forget just how much we matter. We need to take seriously the reality that we are deeply dependent on others for our own sense of value. When others around us treat us as if we are deeply valuable (for example, kind wishes from friends and family on our birthday), we feel ourselves to be valuable. If we are ignored, neglected, forgotten, we quickly begin to doubt our value. Unless we enjoy the respect and dignified treatment of others, we are inclined to feel worthless. In the words of the poet John Donne,

> No man is an island entire of itself; every man
> is a piece of the continent, a part of the main;
> if a clod be washed away by the sea, Europe
> is the less, as well as if a promontory were, as
> well as any manner of thy friends or of thine
> own were; any man's death diminishes me,

because I am involved in mankind.
And therefore never send to know for whom
the bell tolls; it tolls for thee.[8]

None of us is sufficient to establish our own value, independent of the valuations of others. Because others have intrinsic and inherent value, I have an obligation to value them and to communicate that value to them in word and deed. Similarly, they have a responsibility to value me and to communicate that value to me through word and deed. This is the essence of loving community—it is a web of value in action.

To summarize the argument, people really matter, and they ought to be treated accordingly. People have intrinsic value; this is something we recognize. And if they have intrinsic value, then it is necessarily good that they exist. To assert that the existence of something or someone is not necessarily good, or to assert that it is good for someone not to exist, is necessarily to deny that they have intrinsic value. Since assisting suicide expresses the belief that it is good for someone not to exist (it is the act of intentionally causing the person not to exist), it necessarily denies that the person has intrinsic value. As a form of respect for autonomy, assisting suicide appears to value persons, but this is merely a superficial, extrinsic kind of value that does not give us grounds for asserting the intrinsic value of our person. Our autonomy can give rise only to a form of extrinsic value, dependent on our own arbitrary choice as self-valuers. And if we do not intrinsically matter, it's not at all clear why our choices should command the respect of others.

Thus assisting death devalues people. We cannot assist death while also affirming the intrinsic value of that person. As an action, it does not accord with our obligation to treat people as if they really matter. Therefore we ought not to do it.

Christian Insights on Human Value

To this point, I have been arguing from what we may know about the right and the good from nature and reason. Christians refer to such knowledge as a kind of natural (or "general") revelation, something God reveals to us through the created order. To these considerations about human value Christians may add additional knowledge obtained through "special revelation", the Christian Scriptures. Those Scriptures help us to understand intrinsic human value and to appreciate the true depth of that value.

The Bible helps us to understand why people really matter. Above we recognized this value and described it as "intrinsic" to our person, but we never attempted to explain the basis for this value. We know that people really matter, and that is enough for the purposes of the argument about assisted death. Yet understanding where this value comes from is a serious problem in moral philosophy—indeed, the difficulty of explaining how or why we have intrinsic value leads many to deny that we could possibly have it. They are forced to find substitute forms of extrinsic value, such as a reliance on personal autonomy. In our discussion above, we established that personal autonomy is not a sufficient basis for the kind of value that we have.

Special revelation in the Bible gives us a very clear and compelling account of why we are of such value. Genesis 1 tells us that we are made in God's image and likeness. Unique among all the creatures God brought into existence, we alone carry this special status.

In the ancient Near East (i.e., the civilizations of Sumeria, Egypt, etc., that were existent when Genesis was composed), the image of the king was his special representative or envoy. A lesser king would be identified as the image of a greater king whom he served. The image bearer functioned to represent or extend the rule and presence of the greater king; when people saw the lesser king, they would be reminded of the rule and authority of the greater king. A failure to respect the dignity, authority, and honor of the lesser king signified an insult to the greater king. To be created in the image of God, therefore, signifies a special connection to God by virtue of one's role in representing the presence and authority of God within the created sphere.[9]

Moreover, we are created to be godlike in the exercise of dominion over the created order. Equipped with capacities for reason, learning, creativity, ingenuity, language, and speech, we function to continue and expand God's work of creation. Our likeness to God is evident in all our pursuits—architecture, art, music, medicine, science, mathematics, agriculture, engineering, law, carpentry, teaching, storytelling, sailing, and on and on. And in seeing these Godlike capacities and activities in ourselves, we point beyond ourselves to the glory and greatness of our Creator. Just as children remind us of their parents in their behavior and personalities, so when creation sees us, it is to be reminded of God.

Therefore, we are profoundly valuable by virtue of the special role to which we were appointed in creation. It is hard to imagine a position of greater meaning and value.

Throughout the biblical storyline, this sense of value is progressively heightened and celebrated. The psalmist David wondered at the unique value of humanity.

> What is man that you are mindful of him,
>> and the son of man that you care for him?
> Yet you have made him a little lower
>> than the heavenly beings
>> and crowned him with glory and honor.
> You have given him dominion over the works
>> of your hands;
>> you have put all things under his feet.
>
> (Psalm 8:4–6)

The highest demonstration of the true depth of value of each and every individual human is seen in the life, death, and resurrection of Jesus. Jesus devoted himself to communicating value—to caring for the needs of those around him during his ministry, healing the sick, feeding the hungry, restoring outcasts and lepers, befriending the lonely and forsaken, welcoming children, and attending to the spiritual needs of each person he met. The Gospels are remarkable for their stories of Jesus's interactions with individuals. He did not merely value humanity in the abstract; he valued individual people in their concrete lived reality. In his teaching ministry he sought to resolve the many ways in which people had been devalued and to restore our vision of the value of all. Thus he condemned the mistreatment of women, the neglect of the poor, and the fear and loathing of foreigners (Samaritans). The height of hypocrisy, he argued, was to devote oneself to external religious rites to please God while failing to love our neighbor (see the parable of the good Samaritan).

Jesus explicitly taught on human value. The royal commandment, the essence of the good, was to love God and neighbor as we love ourselves. Here, love was understood as value in action, not mere sentiment. In placing the priority of caring for the interests of fellow humans as a close second to the priority of loving and serving God, Jesus implicitly declares the profound value and worth of each and every person. Elsewhere Jesus explicitly speaks of the value that our Heavenly Father places on us.

Therefore I tell you, do not be anxious about your life, what you will eat or what you will drink, nor about your body, what you will put on. ... Look at the birds of the air: they neither sow nor reap nor gather into barns, and yet your heavenly Father feeds them. Are you not of more value than they? And which of you by being anxious can add a single hour to his span of life? And why are you anxious about clothing? Consider the lilies of the field, how they grow: they neither toil nor spin, yet I tell you, even Solomon in all his glory was not arrayed like one of these. But if God so clothes the grass of the field, which today is alive and tomorrow is thrown into the oven, will he not much more clothe you, O you of little faith? Therefore do not be anxious. (Matthew 6:25–31)

Here Jesus combines many truths into a single, concise argument. We need not be anxious for our needs because (1) God is deeply aware of the needs of all living things, (2) God is perfectly capable of meeting our needs with beauty and delight, and (3) we are profoundly valuable in God's sight. In essence, Jesus attributes our tendency to anxiety as the consequence of forgetting just how much we matter to God. He aims to remind us of this deep value and to assure us of God's care. Here he refers to God as our Father—just as a child owns his father's heart, so we enjoy God's paternal delight, devotion, care, and protection. We are so valuable to God that we are like his own children.

The incarnation of the Son of God, Jesus of Nazareth, stands as evidence of the profound value that God places on humanity. In Jesus, God took on human flesh. In becoming man, God declares just how profoundly significant we are, how profoundly important our needs and concerns, and even how precious and valuable are our bodies. Recognizing this, we are exhorted to follow Jesus's example and display the value of others through sacrificial service.

> Let each of you look not only to his own interests, but also to the interests of others. Have this mind among yourselves, which is yours in Christ Jesus, who, though he was in the form of God, did not count equality with God a thing to be grasped, but emptied himself, by taking the form of a servant, being born in the likeness of men. (Philippians 2:4–7)

By entering into the travails of human existence, Jesus demonstrates God's concern for human well-being and our value in his sight. What else could else could more clearly display the exalted status of humanity but that God would become one of us!

In giving his life for us, Jesus demonstrated the depths of our value in God's sight. Jesus submitted himself to suffering and death so that he might atone for our sin and restore us to himself. We see Jesus weeping and groaning in the garden of Gethsemane, and we see how much he loved us and cared for us. We see him rejected, humiliated, subjected to physical and emotional abuse, tortured, and executed, and we see what he was willing to endure in order to take our place and to save us from wrath and condemnation for our insubordination to the Creator's intentions for us. Here the love of God for us—our value in his sight—becomes utterly undeniable.

> For one will scarcely die for a righteous person— though perhaps for a good person one would dare even to die—but God shows his love for us in that while we were still sinners, Christ died for us. (Romans 5:7–8)

> For God so loved the world, that he gave his only Son, that whoever believes in him should not perish but have eternal life. (John 3:16)

> In this the love of God was made manifest among us, that God sent his only Son into the world, so that we might live through him. In this is love, not that we have loved God but that he loved us and sent his Son to be the propitiation for our sins. (1 John 4:9–10)

English physician Thomas Sydenham gave a classic concise summary of the import of the gospel for human value. Addressing the doctor, he wrote, "Let him reflect that he has undertaken the care of no mean creature, for, in order that he may estimate the value, the greatness of the human race, the only begotten Son of God became himself a man, and thus ennobled it with his divine dignity, and far more than this, died to redeem it."[10] The Scripture gives us a vision of the heavenly throngs amazed at what God has done to save and to exalt his treasured people, that people for his own possession who would proclaim the excellencies of his name.

> And they sang a new song, saying,
> "Worthy are you to take the scroll
>   and to open its seals,
> for you were slain, and by your blood you
>   ransomed people for God
>   from every tribe and language and people
>   and nation,
> and you have made them a kingdom
>   and priests to our God,
>   and they shall reign on the earth."
>
> (Revelation 5:9–12)

Thus we come to truly fulfill all that was intended for us as God's image bearers. The true beauty, magnificence, and value of humanity will finally be apparent as priests and kings under God. It is therefore clear that in God's sight, we are priceless and irreplaceable. We have intrinsic value. We really matter.

IV

ASSISTED DEATH IS AN ACT OF SECULAR FAITH

HER TIME HAD come to die. And she knew it. She was looking at me bravely as I came to the bedside. Even though the ventilator was set to deliver high pressures to support her breathing, every breath was now a struggle. Over the preceding weeks, a rare and terrible disease had invaded her lungs, transforming their soft and delicate tissues into hard, rocklike fibers. We had done everything we could, sent every test available, tried multiple treatments in desperation, all to no avail. As her lungs became progressively harder and stiffer, her breathing became more of a struggle, and her oxygen levels dipped lower and lower. We had kept her alive using the mechanical ventilator (breathing machine) to support her breathing and maintain her oxygen levels, but we had come to the point where even the ventilator could no longer inflate her lungs adequately, and there was nothing more to be done. There was now no hope of recovery. It had not been easy to tell her that she was dying. Often when patients are at the limit of life support, they are in a coma, and we are left to break the bad news to the patient's family. But this patient had been wide awake, clear eyed, struggling to breathe, and looking me directly in the eye. She nodded and understood as I told her there was nothing more we could do. She was so very brave.

Since the ventilator was no longer helping her and only prolonging her struggle to breathe, we had decided together to discontinue the breathing machine and let her pass away peacefully and naturally. She had taken time with family to say goodbye, but now she was finding it a severe struggle to go on. The time had come to let her go.

Given the severe damage to her lungs, I told her and her family that she would likely only live for a few minutes after we took her off the breathing machine. As I stood at her bedside, she looked up at me and nodded. She was ready.

We took the breathing tube out and disconnected the ventilator. I knew that every breath would be a struggle, so I gave her a morphine-like drug in repeated steady doses until her breathing was settled and comfortable. I was careful not to give more than I thought was necessary for comfort. She fell asleep. Without the high pressures from the ventilator, her stiff lungs rapidly deflated, and her oxygen levels fell rapidly. She lay in her ICU bed, peacefully dying. Soon she was gone; her struggle was over.

When I left the room, her family was around her body, crying and holding each other. Later, alone in my office, I also wept.

The Uncomfortable Uncertainty of Death

Death is not something we look forward to; it is not something we really like to think about. The fact of death—our own and that of our loved ones—is not a light topic; it's not something we raise casually during polite conversation over dinner. We prefer to ignore it, to speak and to act as if we and those whom we love will always be here. But the fact of our eventual death is there in the background, casting a shadow over all we say and do together.

Sometimes, at the passing of a friend or loved one, we are forced to face up to the reality of death. The grief and shock we experience are difficult to put into words. At one level, we are not surprised by death, for we know that we will all die eventually. Yet, when it comes, death feels very much like a cruel surprise. The dead loved one is truly, actually gone from our midst, never to return. It is inconceivable. And the reality that the same event will come to us in our turn, at some uncertain time in the future, is unsettling. We live much of our lives ignoring the impending reality of our own death and the death of all of those whom we love. Life would be unbearable otherwise.

Why is the idea of death so uncomfortable? Perhaps because it is so final, a point of no return. Perhaps because it presents a final and severe limit on the possibilities of our lives, and forces on us doubts about the meaning and importance of our transient existence. Perhaps death makes us uncomfortable because it presents a great unknown, a horizon over which we cannot see and beyond which we cannot return.

This discomfort over the uncertainty associated with death was expressed by Shakespeare's Hamlet in his famous soliloquy. Contemplating suicide in the face of tragedy, Hamlet longs for deliverance from the travails of life,

> To be, or not to be, that is the question:
> Whether 'tis nobler in the mind to suffer
> The slings and arrows of outrageous fortune,
> Or to take arms against a sea of troubles
> And by opposing end them. To die—to sleep,
> No more; and by a sleep to say we end
> The heart-ache and the thousand natural shocks
> That flesh is heir to: 'tis a consummation
> Devoutly to be wish'd.[11]

In the face of the cruelties of life, only the uncertainty of what lies beyond the grave prevents Hamlet from proceeding to take his own life:

> To die, to sleep;
> To sleep, perchance to dream—ay, there's the rub:
> For in that sleep of death what dreams may come,
> When we have shuffled off this mortal coil,
> Must give us pause—there's the respect
> That makes calamity of so long life ...
> Who would fardels bear,
> To grunt and sweat under a weary life,
> But that the dread of something after death,
> The undiscovere'd country, from whose bourn
> No traveller returns, puzzles the will,

And makes us rather bear those ills we have
Than fly to others that we know not of?[12]

It is the uncertainty of death that prevents him from taking his life—as they say, better the devil you know than the devil you don't.

Over the millennia, humanity has entertained many notions of what happens to us after we die. Every society in human history seems to have had its own particular conception of the afterlife. In the modern era, we mark these theories off as "religions" and regard them as childish stories and fables that we have outgrown. We believe ourselves superior, for we reject superstition and tradition and just-so stories. We require evidence and rely on our direct experience of reality to determine what is real. Our faith is in our conscious brains and our sensory experience—seeing, hearing, touching—to decide what's real. Since dead bodies have no capacity for seeing, hearing, touching, and no brain activity, then dead persons cannot have any experience at all, right? We may have no direct knowledge of what it is like to be dead, but from the incapacity we observe in dead bodies we infer that there is nothing to be experienced. Death, we conclude, is nothingness.

This is the story we tell ourselves. It is a story that manifests deep confidence in the powers of human observation and experience. We deny the possibility that anything could exist that is not accessible to our conscious experience. If we cannot see, touch, or hear it, then it quite simply cannot exist. Absence of evidence, in other words, counts as evidence of absence. It is as if we inhabit a kind of box, the walls of which are defined by human powers of observation and experience. Since, by definition, we cannot sense what lies outside the box, there must be nothing outside the box. The box is the whole story. We live and we die inside the box.

Having accepted this story, we may counsel Shakespeare's Hamlet with more confidence. No need to fear "what dreams may come when we have shuffled off this mortal coil," for we know that there will be no dreams. No need for any "dread of something after death" because there quite simply is no "undiscovered country." As Kurt Vonnegut puts it, "And what is death but an absence of life? That's all it is. That is all it ever can be. Death is nothing. What is all this fuss about?"[13]

Vonnegut made this statement in his famous oration on nuclear weapons in the early 1980s. The speech is titled "Fates Worse than Death." He argued that nuclear disarmament was the only rational course of action because the nuclear arms race put humanity at risk of annihilation, and he could contemplate no realistic fate worse than the death of all humanity (though he made several highly imaginative attempts to do so throughout his speech). These days, talk about "fates worse than death" for individuals is not uncommon, especially in the medical literature[14] in my field of critical care medicine. The rise of powerful life-support technologies can suspend patients in a twilight zone where they require continuous invasive interventions to support life in the absence of any hope of recovery. Some patients who do recover from such life-threatening illnesses are left with substantial permanent physical and cognitive disability. These outcomes—persistent dependence on life support without recovery, or recovery with disability and lasting impairment in quality of life—are sometimes said to be fates worse than death. Of course, these are deeply personal matters. The idea of being worse off alive rather than dead reflects deeply personal values and expectations of what kind of life is worth living. It also professes a confident knowledge of what it is like to be dead, that death is nothing but the absence of life, as Vonnegut put it.

The idea of a fate worse than death helps us to make sense of physician-assisted death. If we can confidently determine that our present state is worse than death, then we may calmly and reasonably decide, in Hamlet's words, to "take arms against a sea of troubles and by opposing, end them." If death is understood to be nothing but the absence of life, the calculus is simply whether the benefits of being alive are outweighed by the harms of being alive. Should the latter outweigh the former, then suicide and physician-assisted death make sense. In such a case, you are better off dead than alive. Death would be good for you.

I do not mean to sound glib. We must not underestimate how attractive death may become when life appears to hold out only frustration, disappointment, and pain. It can be wearisome and exhausting to endure illness and suffering, to bear up against unremitting weakness and progressively worsening physical limitations. Particularly if we are alone, if we do not have support and encouragement from other close friends and caregivers, if we begin to feel that our existence means suffering and hardship for others, if we feel that our existence is only a burden to others, if we cannot see or feel our value, then the thought of death can become truly appealing. Death seems to offer a quiet way out. If death is the absence of life, and life means loneliness, suffering, and hardship, then death seems like peace, rest, and even freedom.

In Death We Trust

We have seen that belief in the benefit of physician-assisted death takes for granted a particular view of death, that death is nothing but the absence of life. If we take this view to be correct, then we can establish whether we are better off dead than alive simply by comparing the benefits and harms of being alive. If the harms of being alive outweigh the benefits, then physician-assisted death is good for us. The death calculus, so to speak, is simply a matter of what it is like to be alive.

Here we encounter a huge problem for those who advocate for physician-assisted death. Put simply, there is no evidence or proof whatsoever to confirm that death is nothing but the absence of life. Indeed, as I will show, reason alone gives us compelling reasons to think that personal existence and consciousness might well continue beyond physical death. And if we cannot take for granted that death is nothing, then we cannot confidently claim that we are better off dead. The death calculus must consider not only what it's like to be alive, but also what it's like to be dead. By our own lights, we have no real way of knowing what it's like to be dead. Given this uncertainty, using death as a remedy for suffering is massively presumptuous, and physician-assisted death is properly viewed as an act of blind faith in death. And because they are willing to lead others to make that leap of blind faith, those who provide physician-assisted death should honestly admit that they are functioning less as doctors and more as priests of a modern, secularized religion that teaches that death is nothing but the absence of life and offers death as the means of salvation from suffering.

Evidence of Absence or Absence of Evidence

Just because you can't see it doesn't mean it's not there.

Think of Anton von Leuwenhoek's discovery of the microscope. Microscopy revealed a whole new world of microscopic organisms that had never been seen or even imagined. Prior to the development of microscopy, some may have wondered about the possibility of cells and microscopic organisms, but there was no strong evidence in support because they couldn't be seen. Yet even before the microscope, it would have been unreasonable (and wrong, in retrospect) to insist that microscopic organisms couldn't possibly exist because they couldn't be seen.

Think of subatomic particles such as the Higgs boson. Peter Higgs proposed that a subatomic particle called a "boson" existed based on mathematical theory long before its existence could be experimentally confirmed. In the decades between Higgs's initial proposal of the existence of this particle and the experiment that confirmed its existence, nobody insisted that it couldn't possibly exist because it had never been detected through human sense experience. This would have been obviously foolish and mistaken.

Sometimes, of course, it is perfectly reasonable to say that something is not there just because it can't be seen. If you say there's somebody standing at the front door and I open the door and don't see anyone, then it's safe for me to say that you are mistaken. The difference, of course, between a Higgs boson and a person standing at the front door is that, in the latter case, I should expect to be able to see them, whereas in the former I would not expect to be able to see it. I can rule out the existence or presence of something by simple eyesight only if simple eyesight can be expected to detect it. More generally, human sense experience can be employed to confirm or refute the existence of something only if that something ought to be detectable by human sense experience.

We see, then, that it is irrational to conclude that there is no life after death simply because we cannot be expected to discover it by sense experience. Our sense experience is confined to the physical, material world defined by space and time, whereas the idea of life after death involves existence beyond that world. While many in our culture deny the possibility of existing outside the material world defined by space and time, they do so only because they have no experience of it. But just because they can't see it or experience it doesn't mean it's not there. Immaterial existence outside space and time is not the kind of thing we would expect to detect by regular human sense experience.

Earlier in the chapter I employed the image of a box that defines the limits of reality based on what is accessible to human sense experience. This box includes all of space-time reality since it is, in principle, detectable by human sense experience (including through microscopes and particle accelerators). All of us find ourselves inside the box. The question is whether there is anything outside the box. To claim that being dead is better than being alive or that death is good for you, you have to insist either that there is nothing outside the box or that you know exactly what is outside the box. And my argument here is simply that we cannot, by sole means of ordinary sense experience, know that there is nothing outside the box or what it is like outside the box.

Death must therefore remain deeply uncertain and mysterious to us, for we have no direct experience of it. Given such uncertainty, we cannot ever assure ourselves that we are better off dead. At some level, ending your life is comparable to leaping off a precipice without knowing what's over the edge. There might be a net to catch you five feet below the edge. Or it might be a very long fall. Relying on ordinary sense experience, we cannot know. And this uncertainty, as Hamlet put it, must give us pause. "There's the respect that makes calamity of so long a life."

Implications for End-of-Life Care

I think it is important for me to offer two clarifying points at this stage in my argument. First, the uncertain nature of death outlined above does not entail that we must do everything possible to stay alive for as long as possible. We are all going to die, even if we are uncertain of what it is like to be dead. When our time comes to die, we don't really have much choice but to accept. As an ICU doctor, I have seen patients or families who struggle to accept the inevitability of death and demand protracted and hopeless life-support interventions. Yet in such cases, delaying death with the use of life support merely serves to prolong suffering in this life without ultimately avoiding the need to face death. My point about the uncertainty of death is not that we should run from death, but rather that we should not claim that death is therapeutic or beneficial. As exemplified in the story I recounted at the outset of this chapter, a palliative philosophy of medical care for patients who are in the final stages of life may wisely accept that death is unavoidable and that medicine may be used to help patients enjoy their remaining days to the fullest extent possible. Such an approach is wise, regardless of the uncertainty of what it is like to be dead. But this approach is very different from actively using death as a remedy for suffering in life. If the nature of death is uncertain, death has no basis for use as a remedy.

This leads to the second point of clarification. The uncertainty of death is of particular importance and relevance for practicing health-care professionals. The uncertainty of death should make the use of death as a remedy for suffering entirely off limits. No responsible doctor or nurse can administer a drug whose effects are completely unknown to them. Because doctors and nurses have no idea what it's like to be dead, causing a patient's death in order to render them better off is akin to starting a patient on experimental therapy and then never following up to see what happens to them. Those who provide assisted death are acting out of blind faith in their own conception of what it is like to be dead. In the absence of medical evidence according to the usual standards, this seems deeply irresponsible.

Let me say a little more on this point. I sometimes hear health-care professionals speak of the benefit of physician-assisted death for patients in terms of the relief of fear and anxiety for patients prior to their death. By offering them control of the timing and manner of dying, some patients feel a sense of relief and freedom. These are undoubtedly important benefits, benefits that could also be largely achieved through assurance of high-quality palliative care through the dying process. What is striking about the notion of benefit here is that it is entirely accrued prior to the administration of any actual intervention. It is the anticipation of death, not the actual death, that is the means of this benefit. To evaluate the benefit of a treatment based on how a patient feels *before* receiving it rather than based on how they feel *after* receiving it is, to put mildly, very unusual.

Put simply, given that it's unknown what happens to patients after they die, it's hard to make out how physician-assisted death can be considered responsible medical practice.

We Think, Therefore We Have an Immaterial Soul

Imagine with me for a moment that humans had both a body and a soul. The body would be the physical aspect of your being, and the soul would be the spiritual or mental aspect of your being. You can think of your soul as being the same thing (more or less) as your mind. If you have such a thing as a soul, then the death of the body would not necessarily mean that your soul was also dead, and it would be, at the very least, possible or plausible for your existence to continue in a disembodied state.

These days most people are taught in school or university to believe that there is no such thing as a soul, primarily because of the widely held belief that science (i.e., the laws of physics and chemistry) can explain everything, including the origin and makeup of humans. A soul, if it were to exist, would have to be something outside the "box"—it is an immaterial substance without dimensions that would exist outside the bounds of space-time reality. If we insist that there is nothing outside the box, there cannot possibly be a soul. If there is no soul, the probability of continued existence beyond physical death would be remote or negligible.

The only problem is that there are actually very good reasons to believe that we have souls simply based on our experience of consciousness and thinking. Let's consider two basic kinds of thinking—reasoning (i.e., thinking about stuff) and willing (i.e., deciding what to think, say, or do). I will argue that these kinds of thinking would not be possible if we did not have a soul. The argument runs as follows: since we "reason" and "will" pretty much continuously while awake, and since we couldn't reason or will if we didn't have a soul, our firsthand, everyday experiences of reasoning and willing give us powerful reasons to believe that we have souls. This in turn gives us a reason to think it quite plausible that human existence could continue beyond bodily death. In this case, death may very well be something different from the mere absence of life.

The Difference between Mind and Brain

We may not immediately appreciate it, but we normally think of and speak of our bodies and our minds as two very different things. Bodily existence and mental existence seem like fundamentally different parts of our experience, even if they are closely and inextricably intertwined. Minds have feelings, thoughts, ideas, beliefs, desires, sensations, and so on, and none of these mental experiences have physical properties, meaning that they can't be described in terms of their location in space and time; they have no dimensions or weight. Nobody else could detect or read our thoughts or feelings through their sense experience. From this standpoint, they appear to exist outside the box of what is accessible to human sense experience. Everything that happens in our bodies, by contrast, is a physical event describable in space and time, through the sciences of biology, chemistry, biochemistry, physics, and biophysics. These events are entirely accessible to human sense experience through measurement, observation, and so on. They all occur inside the box.

Now, many believe that mental experiences (thoughts, feelings, etc.) actually exist inside the box, even though they seem to exist outside the box. In other words, the widely held view is that the mind and mental experience is a kind of illusion produced by that part of the body referred to as the brain. Neuroscientists and philosophers of mind use the term "epiphenomenon," but really this just means "illusion." In this view, the mind and mental activity are nothing more than an apparent by-product of brain function. Mental activity is really just brain activity and is governed by the laws of physics and chemistry just as much as any other part of the body. Mental activity and brain activity are not just correlated; rather, brain activity is the direct and only cause of mental activity. This means that when you are "thinking" you are not really connecting information, ideas, and beliefs together; really, you are experiencing the activity of the brain—the interaction of billions of electrical signals generated within the many highly complex networks of neurons distributed through different parts of the brain. This is really another way of saying that there is nothing outside the box; everything, including the mind, is located within space and time.

Brains Cannot Think (By Themselves)

While we don't often take much time to think about these matters (and I use the term "think" with deliberate irony), it requires only a little thought to realize that attributing your thinking entirely to the activity of your brain results in some really big problems for thinking.

First, you couldn't trust your thought processes (reasoning). The goal of reason is to figure out what is true and not true, what you should believe and what you should not believe. Is the train a reliable way to get to work? Is my English essay due tomorrow? Is this book persuasive? Does this sweater fit me? What's the matter with my brother? Why is there so much suffering in the world? All these questions are constantly running through our heads, and we are constantly thinking and deciding what is true and what is not true. Based on our reason, we form beliefs ("No, this sweater doesn't fit"), and these beliefs determine our actions ("I am going to stop wearing the sweater"). Now suppose that reason is really just neurons firing in response to stimuli from other neurons. Would you have any basis to be confident that neurons firing would produce beliefs that are actually likely to be true? Remember that the firing of neurons is governed by the laws of physics and chemistry, not the laws of logic or evidence. Beliefs are true if they are consistent with logic and evidence, but there is no connection between the laws of logic and the laws of physics and chemistry. If reasoning is really just neurons firing, you would have no basis for confidence that your beliefs are true. In that case, a belief such as "I would be better off dead" would really just be neurons firing, and you cannot be confident that those firing neurons would lead you to the truth. In other words, you can't possibly know that you know anything.

Ironically, this also means that if you believe that everything happens "inside the box" and that thinking is just the firing of neurons, then you would have to doubt whether you could know that was true. It might, in theory, be true that thinking is just the firing of neurons, but you would have no way of proving it or knowing it to be true with any confidence, since you can't rely on neurons to decide between what is true and what is false. They are just cells generating neural outputs in response to other neural inputs.

Of course, I am not saying that brain activity is not necessary for thinking to occur. The point, rather, is that brain activity is not sufficient for thinking to be logical or reliable or trustworthy. If thinking is attributed purely to brain activity, then thinking cannot be trusted.

Brains Do Not Have Free Will

Attributing thinking entirely to brain activity creates a second major problem: you could not have a free will. If thinking were all just brain activity, then all your desires, goals, and decisions would be the consequence of neurons firing. And, since the firing of neurons is completely determined by the laws of physics and chemistry, your desires, goals, and decisions would be entirely controlled by the laws of physics and chemistry. "You" don't decide what you want; rather, physics and chemistry decide. "You" don't control your preferences or goals or values; physics and chemistry control them. "You" don't choose to act; physics and chemistry govern your actions. However much you might feel like "you" are willing and making decisions, it would just be an illusion—it's really just your brain acting according to the laws of nature. This would mean, of course, that you could neither take any credit for good actions or deserve any blame for evil actions (by the way, you also couldn't trust yourself to reliably discern between good and evil, since this requires reason to be reliable and trustworthy).

Biting the Bullet

If you have difficulty accepting these arguments, as straight-forward as they are, don't take it from me. The leading philosophers of our time have pointed out the same thing: if there is no soul, there is no thinking. One leading atheist philosopher writes as follows:

> When I make choices—trivial or momentous—it's just another event in my brain locked into this network of processes going back to the beginning of the universe, long before I had the slightest "choice." Nothing was up to me. Everything—including my choice and my feeling that I can choose freely—was fixed by earlier states of the universe plus the laws of physics. End of story. No free will, just the feeling, the illusion in introspection, that my actions are decided by my conscious will.[15]

This philosopher is totally committed to the idea that everything is inside the box. So he bites the bullet and accepts that since he is only a body and has no soul, therefore he doesn't actually think or have free will. That he decided to write a book with his thoughts on this matter in order to persuade others that they should think the same way is, well, amusing. I hope you can appreciate the irony.

Of course, we really do trust in the reliability of thinking, and we really do believe in free will. The way we live our lives—trusting our thinking, making choices we believe are free, and attributing moral responsibility for choices—shows what we really believe about these points. And if we are to believe that reason and free will are real, then we must affirm the existence of the soul. There really must be something outside the box.

When Arguments Commit Suicide

Astute readers will quickly appreciate that to insist that thinking really happens "inside the box" creates serious difficulties for, among everything else, the case for physician-assisted death.

Physician-assisted death is held to be compassionate and morally good. But if thinking about good and evil is just an illusory by-product of neurons firing, then we wouldn't have any reason to think that our moral judgments are reliable or ought to be believed (since they would not be determined by logic, evidence, and ethics). In that case, we would lose any grounds for claiming that physician-assisted death is morally right or praiseworthy.

Physician-assisted death presumes that patients can reliably think about whether life is worth living, that they can rationally compare the goods of being alive to the evils of being alive, and decide whether death makes sense for them. But if such thinking and reasoning are really just an illusory by-product of neurons firing, such thoughts would be determined by the laws and physics and chemistry, not by logic or evidence or ethics. So, then, we couldn't trust a patient's thought processes (or our own) to decide whether to seek physician-assisted death.

Physician-assisted death presumes that we are in control of our desires and decisions, that we freely and autonomously choose to die. This is a fundamental tenet of the ethical arguments offered to support assisted death; it's all about respect for autonomy. But if our desires and decisions are really just neurons firing under the control of physics and chemistry, then in what sense could we possibly be free in our choice of death? Are "you" choosing death, or are your neurons firing in a pattern that generates an apparent desire for death? And if the latter, do you really have any choice in the matter? Could you desire or choose otherwise? If free will is an impossibility, the idea of autonomy and personal freedom to choose death would collapse. And since the possibility of real personal autonomy is central to the case for physician-assisted death, the case for physician-assisted death would also collapse.

Allow me to sum up the point here. To accept the arguments in support of physician-assisted death, you must believe that thinking, reasoning, and free will are real and not solely governed by physics and chemistry. Yet, as I have shown, belief that thinking and free will are real requires belief that we are not just brains or bodies but also souls.

But belief in the soul requires admission that there is something outside the box and that existence beyond death is a real possibility. Admission that existence beyond death is a real possibility undermines the reliability of judgment that death is good for you (since we no longer know for sure what it is like to be dead). This in turn entails that we don't have any rational basis for deciding whether we benefit from physician-assisted death.

Thus you can't accept the premises underpinning the case for physician-assisted death (real personal autonomy, trustworthiness of our thinking to determine whether death is beneficial) without acquiring a good reason to oppose physician-assisted death (the existence of the soul, hence the plausibility of existence beyond death, hence the uncertainty of the benefit of death). In this way, we see that the case for physician-assisted death is actually self-refuting.

Science or Religion?

I do not mean to suggest that everyone who supports physician-assisted death believes that death is nothing. Social science and health services research studies have consistently shown a strong correlation between a lack of (formal) religious belief and support for the practice—those who profess to be nonreligious are much more likely to support physician-assisted death, while those who profess devout commitment to the traditional monotheistic religious belief systems (Christianity, Islam, Judaism) are more likely to oppose it. Yet some people who support physician-assisted death may profess religious or spiritual beliefs, including belief in life beyond death of some kind, whether in heaven or through reincarnation. I imagine that many of those who support physician-assisted death might not insist that there is nothing outside the box.

Regardless of what you believe about life after death (or the absence thereof), my point simply is that your belief about what it is like to be dead is necessarily engaged when you decide that death could be good for you. Put differently, you cannot decide whether it would be good to exit the box without forming some opinion as to what is outside the box. If you don't know what's out there, you simply have no way of knowing whether death is good for you.

Support for physician-assisted death, therefore, relies on your beliefs about the afterlife, whatever they might be. In this sense, physician-assisted death is an act of faith. When we use death to escape the hardships of this life, we presume to know what death is like. Because those who claim that death is nothing don't really know that for sure, physician-assisted death is best considered an act of blind faith on their part. It is an act at least as superstitious and religious as any carried out in any religious services of any kind. Those who administer physician-assisted death are functioning not as doctors but as priests, helping their patients by ushering them out of life and into the afterlife, the great unknown.

Christian Perspective on Death

Christianity recognizes death as the central problem of our existence. Or to put it more precisely, Christianity understands death to be the primary symptom of the central problem of our existence. That problem is our separation from God by virtue of humanity's shared rebellion against God's authority. We were created to be God's children, made in his image and likeness. Like foolish and disobedient children, we insist on having our way and making our own rules. We seek happiness not in knowing and serving our Father but instead in some aspect of his creation—money, fame, sexual pleasure, friendships, accomplishments. All these are good things, but they are not worthy of being that for which we live primarily. And in worshiping ourselves and the things God created rather than God himself (an act called idolatry), we have fractured our relationship to God and cut ourselves off from fellowship with him. The consequence of this is death. Physical death is a sign of spiritual death. Physical death is the hard and shocking evidence of the futility of our existence apart from life in God.

Our rejection of God is exemplified in our rejection of Jesus. He had the audacity to declare that he was the Son of God, the Son of Man, the long-awaited Messiah, the Savior of the world, the only way to God. The truthfulness of that claim was confirmed by many lines of evidence: the fulfillment of many prophecies about who the Messiah would be, where he would be born, and how he would live, suffer, die, and rise from the dead; his countless miracles of healing and demonstrations of power over nature, powers always used for the good of others around him; the beauty and divinity of his teaching matched only by the beauty and divinity of his life.

But the greatest proof of Jesus's divinity is his resurrection from the dead. Jesus himself forewarned his disciples on multiple occasions that he would be crucified in Jerusalem and would rise again from the dead. Knowing these predictions, his enemies sought a Roman guard to watch over his tomb after his death and burial so that nobody could steal his body away and claim that he had been resurrected. Yet, two days later his body was missing from the tomb, and multiple people began to report different sightings and encounters with Jesus, so much so that they became convinced that he was risen from the dead. According to some witnesses, he appeared to over five hundred people at once at one point. Those who witnessed his bodily appearances were so convinced of his resurrection that they were willing to suffer and die for their faith in Jesus. On this basis, Christians are convinced that Jesus was resurrected from the dead.[16] By his resurrection, Jesus vindicated his authority to speak on matters of life and death and achieved a complete and entire victory over our ultimate enemy, death itself.

In Death, Christians Anticipate True Life

For Christians, death is neither uncertain nor fearful. We worship a man who returned from the dead with a guarantee of resurrection and eternal life for those who follow him in faith and obedience. The night before Jesus was crucified he promised, "In my Father's house are many rooms. If it were not so, would I have told you that I go to prepare place a for you? And if I go and prepare a place for you, I will come again and will take you to myself, that where I am you may be also. And you know the way to where I am going" (John 14:2–4).

For those who have followed the Way, death is the way to life, true life in the company of the one who loved us and gave himself for us. Indeed, we believe we are united with him in his death and resurrection: our spiritual reality is that we have died with him and we have been raised with him. This reality is signified powerfully in Christian baptism: "having been buried with him in baptism, in which you were also raised with him through faith in the powerful working of God, who raised him from the dead" (Colossians 2:12). In Jesus, we have already died: "For you have died, and your life is hidden with Christ in God. When Christ who is your life appears, then you also will appear with him in glory" (Colossians 3:3–4). In Jesus, we have stared death in the face, and it stands defeated. We may die, but then we will live, and truly live. For we will live eternally in the presence of God without any sense of limitation or impending end to life.

> When the perishable puts on the imperishable, and the mortal puts on immortality, then shall come to pass the saying that is written:

> "Death is swallowed up in victory."
> "O death, where is your victory?
>   O death, where is your sting?"
>   (1 Corinthians 15:53)

For Christians, death is life. It is our entrance into glory. It is the means by which we enter into that which "no eye has not seen, nor ear heard, nor the heart of man imagined, what God has prepared for those who love him" (1 Corinthians 2:9). Thus Paul the apostle professed that he longed "to depart and be with Christ, for that is far better" (Philippians 1:23).

Here Paul explicitly gives us his own death calculus. Through the testimony of Jesus Christ, Paul knows what it is like to be dead. It is an incomparable and eternal weight of glory (2 Corinthians 4:17). If Paul were to weigh up the goods and evils of remaining alive and set these alongside the good of departing to be with Christ, there would be no comparison. The calculus was vastly in favor of preferring death to life. Thus he declares that "my desire is to depart and be with Christ, for that is far better." "To live is Christ," he says, "and to die is gain" (Philippians 1:21).

So we arrive at a remarkable apparent paradox. Christians confidently believe that they are better off dead, yet they refuse to use death as an escape from suffering (i.e., physician-assisted death). How can we make sense of this? Why do we remain to bear the slings and arrows of cruel fortune? If we really believe with Paul that death is gain, then why don't we take matters into our own hands to end things now and enter into the glory that awaits us?

We saw part of the answer in the previous chapter—our intrinsic and incalculable value makes us untouchable, even to ourselves. Destroying something devalues it; out of recognition of our intrinsic value, we must not and cannot destroy ourselves. We turn now to consider another part of the answer: the possibility that even in the face of irremediable suffering, our existence has unassailable purpose, meaning, and significance.

V

Escape
from Despair

I N THIS BOOK, I set out to answer the "Why not?" question regarding physician-assisted death. We saw that intentionally causing someone's death contravenes and violates their intrinsic and incalculable worth. So long as we are committed to upholding the intrinsic value of persons—so long as we insist that their value does not merely derive from their usefulness to others or to themselves—it is inappropriate and unethical for us to seek or to offer physician-assisted death. We also saw that relying on our own sense experience and human faculties, we cannot confidently claim to know what it is like to be dead. Therefore, it is unwise and imprudent to seek and (especially) to offer physician-assisted death.

These reasons, I think, count quite strongly against physician-assisted death. It certainly seems like we have a very good answer to the "Why not?" question. Is the case then closed? Not quite, I think. For to respond effectively to this issue, we must not only address the "Why not?" question. We must also respond to the "Why?" question. We must address the deep, underlying motivation for seeking or offering physician-assisted death. We must face the suffering of the sufferer, and we must have something better to offer than death.

Michael's Story

When I met Michael, he was about thirty years old. I was a young medical student, learning how to take the patient's history and perform a physical examination. He was the patient, admitted to the hospital for a urinary tract infection. This particular admission for a urinary tract infection was just one of many previous such admissions. Michael had primary progressive multiple sclerosis. He could barely move his arms and legs; they were stiff and contracted. He was blind. I recall peering with my ophthalmoscope into his unseeing eyes, the white plaques of optical neuritis from multiple sclerosis effacing the surface of the retina. With the loss of some spinal cord functions, his bladder no longer contracted. To prevent urinary retention, he had an indwelling urinary catheter, but this was also a conduit for repeated infection. These infections left him much weaker even than normal, prostrate in bed, nauseated, in pain, and profoundly unwell.

As a young medical student, his condition made a striking impression of suffering and disability. I had not encountered many people with such severe chronic illness to that point. My world had been walled off from that of people like him. I lived with my new wife in our comfortable apartment; he lived in his nursing home. I was surrounded by friends and family; he was alone. I came and went as I pleased; he was bedbound. My future was that of expanding skill and opportunity. His future held out progressively increasing discomfort and limitation. In that hospital room, our worlds collided. I was the doctor-in-training; he was the lesson. But we were also just two young men struggling to find our way in the world.

Michael was shrouded in despair. He was diagnosed with multiple sclerosis as an older teenager. The disease had progressively taken away his abilities and liberties; it had stolen everything a young man dreams of in life. Now, a decade later, he was desperately alone and desperately sad. He was deeply lonely; his disease had cut him off from friendship. It was not for lack of interest on his part, though friendship under such circumstances was undoubtedly difficult. Perhaps it was too easy for others to forget about him; perhaps it was too uncomfortable to visit. After all, when we see such suffering we feel threatened, for we are tempted by a vague horror that the same might happen to us. Only with the kind of repeated exposure to suffering and disease that medical students and residents experience during their training can one develop the disciplined sense of invulnerability necessary to cope (though this can also be profoundly unhealthy).

His loneliness was compounded by profound hopelessness. His was a progressive disease, unrelenting in its attack on his brain and spinal cord. His future held no hope for meaningful improvement, no possibility of freedom or relief. He spoke of the struggle to get through the day, feeling that there was little point in going on. What was the purpose, the meaning, the point of such a life? It was gut wrenching for me to sit and listen. I felt the cruelty and injustice of the world. "Why him? Why not me?" I thought.

Our clinical encounter was soon finished. I left, profoundly moved by his suffering. For a brief moment I had the privilege of seeing the world through his eyes. I could sense his struggle to keep from coming apart and to retain his sense of personhood and dignity in the face of his disability and suffering. He was mourning a deep sense of loneliness, pointlessness, and hopelessness. His battle for survival was a battle with despair.

Grappling with Despair

The desire for physician-assisted death should be understood as a cry of despair, a cry that cannot be ignored. To ignore that cry denies the worth and value of the sufferer just as much as causing their death denies that value. Imagine for a moment that you are walking near the edge of a cliff and you hear a distress cry at the edge. Looking over the edge, you see someone clinging to a ledge, hanging precariously and desperately fearful of plunging to the rocks below. Suppose a friend who is with you offers them a high dose of fast-acting sleeping medicine to help them fall asleep so they no longer experience fear or distress. You might successfully convince both your friend and the person whose life is in danger that it would be unhelpful, unwise, and inappropriate to offer or ingest the sleeping medicine. But the problem remains—how do you actually help them in their moment of peril?

Likewise, even if we have successfully shown that physician-assisted death is an inappropriate and unwise way to respond to suffering, our task is not complete. We have failed to truly care for our patients if we hear their cries of despair, their requests for death, and simply throw our hands up to say, "Sorry, it's wrong for me to end you, so I can't help you." Rather, we must probe the reasons for the request; we must understand the fears and the pain that lead to such a cry. And we must find a way to come to their aid. It remains to us to offer a better way for our fellow humans who find themselves in the crucible of suffering.

In many ways, an effective response to the "Why?" question would render the "Why not?" question moot. If we can show that physician-assisted death is unnecessary in the first place, if we can show how we may bear the unbearable, then we have gone a very long way to resolving the issue. Answers to the "Why not?" question are thus really secondary to finding a deep solution for the "Why?" question.

What, then, is that solution? How do we help others to bear their suffering? Is there an escape from despair?

Finding a Reason to Live

Nietzsche, always an incisive observer of the human condition, was quoted to say that "he who has a 'why' to live can bear almost any 'how.'"[17] Lacking the why—the sense of a point to one's existence and one's suffering—the how may become unbearable. We humans hunger for meaning; starved of it, we die. Without meaning and purpose, our existence feels futile, absurd, and intolerable. French existentialist playwright and philosopher Albert Camus famously declared, "There is but one truly serious philosophical problem, and that is suicide." By this he meant that "judging whether life is or is not worth living amounts to answer the fundamental question of philosophy."[18] For what reason do we struggle on against the "slings and arrows of outrageous fortune"? Why not simply make a quiet exit? For some reason, we want to live, though we can't always understand why.

Few have written of the deep human need for meaning and purpose with more penetrating insight than Viktor Frankl. Frankl was a Jewish psychiatrist who endured the horrors of several Nazi concentration camps during World War II. Frankl's parents, wife, and brother died in the camps at the hands of the Nazis; he alone survived. Frankl wrote movingly of his experiences of the Holocaust in a global bestseller titled *Man's Search for Meaning*. In that work, Frankl recounts the power of meaning to endure unthinkable suffering. He came to believe that his survival in the camps and that of his fellow prisoners depended on finding some purpose for their existence, even as their Nazi captors did everything possible to make their lives seem utterly pointless and unendurable. Meaning, he argues, is essential for survival.

> Any attempt to restore a man's inner strength in the camp had first to succeed in showing some future

goal. Nietzsche's words, "He who has a why to live can bear almost any how," could be the guiding motto for all [mental health] efforts regarding prisoners. Whenever there was an opportunity for it, one had to give them a why—an aim—for their lives, in order to strengthen them to bear the terrible how of their existence. Woe to him who saw no more sense in his life, no aim, no purpose, and therefore no point in carrying on. He was soon lost.[19]

Frankl emphasized the deadly consequences of loss of meaning. "Those who know how close the connection is between the state of mind of a man—his courage and hope, or lack of them—and the state of immunity of his body will understand that the sudden loss of hope and courage can have a deadly effect."[20] Frankl went on to establish an influential school of psychotherapy that employed the discovery of meaning (he referred to it as logotherapy) as the basis for restoring and maintaining mental health.

Frankl was not alone in his observations. Eminent Canadian psychiatrist and palliative care researcher Harvey Max Chochinov described the central role that meaning and purpose play in upholding a sense of personal dignity for patients with terminal illness. He and his team interviewed over two hundred patients at the end of life admitted to palliative care units, inquiring about the factors that affected their sense of personal dignity in the face of their impending death.[21] The patients identified key factors that impaired their sense of dignity, factors such as being treated disrespectfully, feeling burdensome, losing control of life, or feeling a lack of a lasting contribution to the world. Of all the concerns raised, the factor that best predicted loss of dignity was "feeling life no longer has a meaning or purpose." The authors conclude, "Clearly, engendering a sense of meaning or purpose, as a way of staving off feelings of being a burden and no longer feeling worthy of respect, is a cornerstone of dignity conserving care." This research bears out Frankl's observations of those struggling to live in the face of death. The instinct to live and the desire for life depend on a sense of meaning and purpose.

Creating Meaning Out of Nothing

How, then, do we find meaning and purpose to sustain our desire for life in the face of suffering? This is the fundamental problem of pain. What kind of meaning and purpose could make a life of pain and suffering worth living?

Christian author and Pastor Tim Keller helpfully distinguished between two different kinds of meaning.[22] There is what he termed created meaning—meaning that we create for ourselves through our endeavors and pursuits. We set a goal for ourselves, and the journey to the fulfillment of this goal becomes a source of meaning in our life. We can have many such meanings at once, some of them simple and short term, some of them ambitious and long term. Such sources of meaning might include our career and related accomplishments, our relationships with family and friends, sexual pleasure, travel, writing, reading, sports, or religion and spiritual interests. Through these meanings, our lives come to feel meaningful, and the effort to see these meanings fulfilled makes life worth living to us.

The unifying feature of created sources of meaning is that they are chosen or produced by us, not given to us. They are self-created. They become my meaning if and only if I adopt them to be my meaning. In no sense is such meaning given or assigned to me by someone else. Such meaning becomes mine in the same way that an item of clothing becomes mine as I choose to make a retail purchase. This way of thinking about meaning reflects a kind of consumer mentality about meaning and purpose—I choose my meaning from many options. Once I choose, the meaning becomes my meaning, but not until then. It is in this sense that Keller says that we create our meaning(s).

This kind of meaning, self-created meaning, is how many people think about the meaning of their life. In a survey study, Canadian psychologist David Speed found that very few people affirmed the statement "Life does not serve any purpose."[23] On the other hand, many affirmed the statement "Life is only meaningful if you provide the meaning yourself." These people, mostly nonreligious, looked for meaning from within rather than from outside. They affirmed self-created meaning.

The Unbearable Burden of
Self-Created Meaning

But the problem of meaning is not so easily solved. If the creation of my meaning depends on me, then the sustaining of my meaning also depends on me. Any given possible meaning becomes my meaning only so long as I continue to own it and only so long as I find it meaningful. But meanings, like clothes, wear thin and wear out over time. We might, for example, find that work no longer brings a sense of meaning the way it once did. So we seek meaning elsewhere, in other pursuits, in new relationships, in new challenges. If circumstances change such that a particular goal or pursuit becomes unavailable to us—you discover that you will never climb through an organization as you had hoped you might— then that particular goal or pursuit can no longer serve to make your life meaningful. Since you are unable to sustain that source of meaning as meaningful, you lose your meaning until you can find it elsewhere. These experiences can be devastating, emotionally, psychologically, and spiritually.

The fundamental barrier to sustaining self-created sources of meaning is that we are limited. We are limited in what we can accomplish and engineer in our life despite our best efforts at taking control. In our pursuit of meaningful purposes and goals, we may be stymied and we may fail. Those purposes and goals can no longer continue to give us meaning, even if they served us well for a time. Our story will need to be about something else.

We are also limited in lifespan. If our chosen sources of meaning depend on us for their continued significance, then they cannot possibly outlast us. After we are gone, others cannot look back and say that our lives mattered because of *x* source of meaning. Rather, they can only say that our lives mattered *to us at the time* because of *x* source of meaning. If our meaning and purpose are self-created and self-defined, then they die with us.

Suffering and dying provoke despair because it is hard for us to sustain any sense of meaning and purpose in the face of pain that, at bottom, seems pointless. Suffering makes it hard for us to create meaning for ourselves, because we cannot avoid the grim reality that self-created meaning is really only a pleasant fiction. When life is pleasurable, we can distract ourselves from our meaningless with self-created meaning. But when we suffer, distraction is no longer possible. Leo Tolstoy writes, "It is possible to live only as long as life intoxicates us; as soon as we are sober again we see that it is all a delusion, and a stupid one."[24] Life and its pursuits and its self-created meanings serve to distract us from the real emptiness and brevity of life. But once one is sobered up by suffering, it is harder to avoid the emptiness of life. Suffering puts pressure on all our sources of meaning; unless meaning and purpose can be sustained in the face of suffering, we are forced to despair.

Physician-assisted death is held up as a solution to the problem of suffering; at bottom, it is really an act of despair.

Choosing death makes sense when life feels pointless. Albert Camus understood the intuitive link between despair and suicide. "Dying voluntarily implies that you have recognized, even instinctively ... the absence of any profound reason for living, the insane character of that daily agitation [of bearing with suffering and trouble], and the uselessness of suffering."[25] Blunt words, but honest. Camus puts it so well: suffering seems useless.

In an earlier chapter, we were introduced to Gillian Bennett, the woman who took her own life following her diagnosis of Alzheimer's dementia. Camus's assertion that suffering is useless strongly echoes through her own words:

> Understand that I am giving up nothing by committing suicide. All I lose is an indefinite number of years of being a vegetable in a hospital setting, eating up the country's money but having not the faintest idea of who I am. ... Nurses, who thought they were embarked on a career that had great meaning, find themselves perpetually changing my diapers and reporting on the physical changes of an empty husk. It is ludicrous, wasteful, and unfair.

Not only was her suffering useless, but she felt that she herself would be useless. The pointlessness of life robbed her of significance and value as a person. The thought of being a burden, of robbing others of meaning and value in their life, was abhorrent to this brilliant and articulate woman.

Death for her was a courageous act of self-extinction that held out freedom from absurdity for her and for those who would have been called on to care for her. Death was her escape from despair.

Real Meaning

Keller identifies a second kind of meaning, which he refers to as discovered meaning. This kind of meaning is "meaning that is there, apart from your feelings or interpretations."[26] Unlike self-created meaning, which comes from within, discovered meaning is outside us, above and beyond us. It is a meaning that is simply given to us, apart from our choice. If such meaning were to exist, it would be our actual meaning, whether we discover it or not. With self-created meaning, we are like a blank notebook, waiting to be given a story. With discovered meaning, we are like a book where the words are already written. To find out what we are about, our task is simply to read the words already there.

Keller points out that discovered meaning is more durable than self-created meaning. Discovered meaning is not affected by circumstance or fortune. It outlasts and transcends us. Such meaning, if it can be found, sustains us through adversity; it does not rely on us to be sustained. If we have discovered a meaning "out there," if our story is being written for us, then suffering and dying cannot rob us of meaning and purpose. Indeed, suffering may become profoundly meaningful insofar as it achieves some higher and lasting good and advances some larger purpose that transcends our own brief period of existence. If our suffering is part of some larger story, a story in which everything is ultimately brought together for good, and if that story is true, then our suffering and our dying could even be worth it, in the end. Surely nothing could be more profoundly valuable than the discovery of such a meaning for our existence.

In our cultural moment, most people are deeply skeptical about the possibility of discovering true meaning. It just seems implausible to them, given the way that they naturally regard the world. To talk about true meaning is like talking about a story with a fairytale ending—it just seems too good to be true, like something we should not even bother hoping for. Real meaning—discovered meaning—seems to elude our grasp; it is something beyond our reach.

Perhaps the most important cause of this skepticism about meaning is the "death of God" in our culture. The widespread attitude that God does not exist or that his existence cannot really be known or confirmed undermines any basis for discovered meaning. How so? Put simply, every story needs an author. If we deny the existence of an Author of our lives, then life is a blank notebook awaiting a story rather than a story already written and waiting to be read. If there is no Author, then there is no grand, overarching story, and we are left to play author on that blank notebook, each writing our own story and crafting our own narrative. The denial of God is at once liberating—we write our own story—and profoundly terrifying, for we are left in despair and absurdity. Our stories are nothing more than wishful thinking, "a tale that is told, full of sound and fury, signifying nothing."[27]

Mathematician and philosopher Bertrand Russell was brutally honest about the consequences of rejecting the Author for the possibility of meaning. In his famous essay *A Free Man's Worship* he writes,

> That Man is the product of causes which had no prevision of the end they were achieving; that his origin, his growth, his hopes and fears, his loves and his beliefs, are but the outcome of accidental collocations of atoms; that no fire, no heroism, no intensity of thought and feeling, can preserve an individual life beyond the grave; that all the labours of the ages, all the devotion, all the inspiration, all the noonday brightness of human genius, are destined to extinction in the vast death of the solar system, and that the whole temple of Man's achievement must inevitably be buried beneath the debris of a universe in ruins—all these things, if not quite beyond dispute, are yet so nearly certain, that no philosophy which rejects them can hope to stand. Only within the scaffolding of these truths, only on the firm foundation of unyielding despair, can the soul's habitation henceforth be safely built.[28]

Despair—unyielding despair—is the inevitable and necessary consequence of excluding God. Many around us feel compelled to exclude God because they do not know how belief in God can be rationally accepted, and they find themselves preferring the freedom of self-created meaning to the constraints of discovered meaning. Then, when suffering leaves our self-created meanings feeling thin and empty, the firm foundation of unyielding despair is uncovered.

Glimmers of Real Meaning
Are All around Us

Though the possibility of discovering real meaning seems dim in our cultural moment, it has not been fully extinguished. We may feel like sailors adrift at sea on a foggy night, hopeless of finding our port of call, our place of belonging. Yet if we strain our eyes searchingly through the murky darkness, we can catch glimmers of the light. For the signs of meaning are all around for us to see, if we will but open our eyes. We have become so accustomed to building our life on a foundation of unyielding despair that we are almost reluctant to give up the project. Could we have been wrong all this time? It seems too much to allow our hearts to hope. And yet, I say, there are glimmers. Upon studied reflection, they grow brighter and brighter.

If there is something in the world that really matters, something genuinely valuable and significant, then discovered meaning must be possible. And we are that something.

As we saw in chapter 2, we have intrinsic and incalculable value. We matter, and not merely because we are useful to ourselves or to others. We may not be able to explain why we matter, but we know we matter, for we see the evil of mistreating others and of mistreatment against ourselves. This means that good and evil are really real. They are not something we imagine or create. They are there. By promoting the good and obstructing the evil, by valuing our neighbor according to the true depth of their value through our words and actions, by making their interests our own, we participate in a good that is bigger and more durable than ourselves. In loving our neighbors, we discover real meaning for our lives.

Moreover, because we have intrinsic value, it is good that we exist. Our existence is good, in and of itself. The intrinsic goodness of our existence means that our existence matters. Merely by virtue of our existence, the world is a better place. The meaning of our lives is literally built into our very existence, no matter our circumstances or limitations. Inclined as we are to evaluate ourselves in terms of our impact, to struggle for worth and value through our deeds and accomplishments, we doubt that mere existence is enough for meaning. Yet, if we have intrinsic value, then our existence matters, apart from any of our deeds. The cosmos is a better place simply because we are here. Thank you for being here.

Nature itself betrays bright glimmers of meaning, if we will but look. What is beauty in nature but the sign of an intrinsic goodness to be promoted and celebrated staring us in the face? What is the Big Bang, the onset of space and time, but the work of an Author commencing a story? Nothing comes from nothing. What is the fine-tuning of the cosmos but the hand of a Designer behind our existence? What is information in genetic material but the hand of that same Designer? Design and purpose are literally in our DNA. We're not here by accident, and the evidence of a purpose behind our existence is not subtle.[29]

In chapter 3 we saw that we are not just bodies but also souls. Our bodies, governed as they are by the laws of physics and chemistry, have no capacity for genuine creative freedom. Yet we are in fact genuinely creative. (Indeed, we exercise this creative freedom in adopting self-created meanings.) Therefore, we are more than just bodies governed by the laws of nature; we are also minds with capacity for thought, knowledge, and free exercise of our will. And if we are more than bodies, then we are more than what nature could generate. Nature, limited to space and time, cannot give rise to the immaterial. The impersonal cannot give rise to the personal. If we see in ourselves the capacity for genuine self-authoring, then we must have an Author from whom this capacity derives. Nature, impersonal and material as it is, could not grant us this capacity.[30] And if we have an Author, then we have a story waiting to be read. We have a meaning waiting to be discovered.

Good News for Those Hungry for Meaning

Jesus taught, "The kingdom of heaven is like treasure hidden in a field, which a man found and covered up. Then in his joy he goes and sells all that he has and buys that field. Again, the kingdom of heaven is like a merchant in search of fine pearls, who, on finding one pearl of great value, went and sold all that he had and bought it" (Matthew 13:44–46). Participation in the kingdom of God, in other words, is of incomparable value. It has something to offer us that we cannot find elsewhere. The discovery of this treasure leaves us willing to sell everything else. Without the kingdom, we might as well have nothing. With the kingdom, we have everything.

What is it about the kingdom that is of such profound value? It is a multifaceted treasure, but at the center of its value is the possibility of ultimate meaning. Jesus's gospel of the kingdom is good news because it offers us deep, durable meaning powerful enough to sustain us through life and through suffering and dying. Our story becomes part of God's grand story, the story behind all of our stories. It is the story in which our suffering is shown to be for good, to be meaningful, to matter, to be worth it. And it is a happily-ever-after story, a too-good-to-be-true story, a story of faith, hope, and love that culminates in eternal life and everlasting communion with the One who made us for himself. In the kingdom, we discover that God himself is our highest good. In the kingdom, we discover a meaning for our suffering that makes it all worth it. In the kingdom, our suffering is not useless. In the kingdom, there is no despair.

Jesus Confronts Suffering

How, then, does the gospel enable us to bear up in the face of suffering and to find meaning in the midst of our pain? To explore this, we turn to the story of Lazarus recorded in John's Gospel (John 11). Lazarus was a dear friend of Jesus and beloved brother to Mary and Martha. Jesus loved this family and visited them often. When Lazarus fell seriously ill, his sisters hastened to contact Jesus to ask him to come and to heal him. They knew of his healing ministry and had confidence that he could restore Lazarus to health. Yet strangely, despite his professed love for Lazarus, Jesus delayed. Before he finally arrived, Lazarus died. Indeed, Lazarus was in the tomb for four days by the time he arrived. Mary, Martha, and the entire community were devastated. They could not understand why Jesus would delay coming to save such a close friend. Martha and Mary separately expressed their grief and consternation with the same words. "Lord, if you had been here, my brother would not have died" (John 11:21).

Jesus's response to their pain, both his words and his actions, teaches us to see suffering as meaningful and worthwhile. He shows them—and us—that suffering is not pointless. Our suffering matters because our story fits into a bigger story, a story that he is bringing together toward a happy and satisfying ending. Through suffering, we see more clearly our need for God, and we discover meaning and satisfaction in God himself. Pain is never good in and of itself, but when we discover the true meaning of our pain, we may transcend our pain, and thereby we may endure it with patience and joy. We can explore Jesus's response to their pain through the rubric of faith, hope, and love.

Patient Endurance through Faith in Christ

Jesus responds to their pain with an invitation to trust in God's purposes and power. Unbeknownst to Martha and Mary, he already declared to his disciples that Lazarus's death and their suffering have a deep purpose. "This illness does not lead to death. It is for the glory of God, so that the Son of God may be glorified through it" (John 11:4). Later, as they are journeying to see the family, Jesus tells his disciples, "Lazarus has died, and for your sake I am glad that I was not there, so that you may believe" (11:14). These sayings of Jesus must have seemed cryptic to the disciples. How could Lazarus's suffering bring glory to the Son of God (a term by which Jesus refers to himself)? How would Lazarus's death become the reason for deepening faith and belief in Jesus? Indeed, their response reveals a kind of resignation and hopelessness on their part about a journey that will take them near Jerusalem. Thomas, later called Doubting Thomas, "said to his fellow disciples, 'Let us also go, that we may die with him'" (11:16).

On Jesus's arrival, Martha professes her faith in Jesus. "Lord, if you had been here, my brother would not have died. But even now I know that whatever you ask from God, God will give you" (11:21). But as they proceed to the graveside, and Jesus makes the shocking request to "Take away the stone," Martha's doubts quickly become apparent. "Lord, by this time there will be an odor, for he has been dead four days" (11:39). Jesus's rebuke is gentle. "Did I not tell you that if you believed you would see the glory of God?" (11:40).

Bystanders also express their doubt about Jesus's power and purposes. "Could not he who opened the eyes of the blind man also have kept this man from dying?" (11:37). It did not occur to them that Jesus has the power to bring life even those who have died. Their limited confidence in his power leaves them mystified as to his purposes: Why didn't he intervene to keep him from dying?

The challenge of suffering is to believe that God's power and purposes are adequate to make our suffering make sense. Pain feels pointless to the extent that we doubt God. But where faith grows strong, despair dies. Through his actions—indeed, through all of Scripture—Jesus gives us abundant reasons to trust his power and purposes.

Jesus proceeds to vindicate his own power and purposes by raising Lazarus from the dead. It becomes clear that he allowed Lazarus to suffer and to die just so that others could see something they could not otherwise have seen. Before raising Lazarus, Jesus prays aloud that "they may believe that you sent me." And then "he cried out with a loud voice, 'Lazarus, come out'" (11:43). Moments later, the dead man emerges, wrapped in his funeral shroud and embalming cloths. Lazarus is alive. The effect is exactly that for which Jesus aimed. "Many of the Jews therefore, who had come with Mary and had seen what he did, believed in him" (11:45). The magnitude of God's power and the beauty of his purposes are put on full display, and Jesus's audience suddenly finds faith to be irresistible.

Confident Joy through Hope in Christ

Jesus also responds to their pain with an invitation to hope. Suffering produces despair by leaving us hopeless of a better future, but Jesus's words and actions invite Martha and Mary to hope for the possibility of something better than their present pain. Speaking of Lazarus's death, Jesus tells his disciples, "Our friend Lazarus has fallen asleep, but I go to awaken him" (11:11). To call death sleep is to reject its finality. When Martha expresses her grief and despair to Jesus, Jesus responds, "Your brother will rise again" (11:23). When Martha expresses her assent to this belief (not universal among the Jews at the time), Jesus invites her to put her hope specifically in him. "I am the resurrection and the life. Whoever believes in me, though he die, yet shall he live, and everyone who lives and believes in me shall never die. Do you believe this?" (11:25–26). Throughout the Gospel of John, Jesus is repeatedly recorded as offering eternal life through faith in him. By casting ourselves on him, recognizing his lordship, and submitting ourselves to following him, we have hope of a future existence absolutely free of any suffering, dying, grief, and despair. Death is our final enemy, our deepest limit, the ultimate reason for despair. In Jesus, death has been conquered, and the possibility of freedom from death is on offer to "whoever believes in me."

Illness, pain, suffering, and dying may cast their shadow over us for a time. But it is only for a time. They make us feel limited, but in Jesus they have become limited. They can no longer drive us to despair, for we have sure and certain hope of final victory over death. Nothing about our pain takes Jesus by surprise. He is fully aware and fully in control. He knows how to bring our stories—knit together with God's story as the true story—to a happy ending. Jesus vindicated that hope by raising Lazarus from the dead, and not many days hence he himself was raised from the dead in a glorious demonstration of his final victory over death. Sooner than we expect, we too will be raised with him in glory (Colossians 3:1–4). In the midst of our pain, in Jesus we find hope of a future free of suffering and of everlasting rest. Augustine expresses that hope in stirring prose at the close of his massive *City of God*: "There we shall rest and see, see and love, love and praise. Behold what will be, in the end to which there shall be no end! For what other end do we set for ourselves than to reach that kingdom of which there is no end?"[31]

Satisfaction and Rest in the Love of Christ

But before this end comes, in the here and now, we must suffer. Yet we do not suffer alone. In one of the most moving moments recorded in the Gospels, we see Jesus's own grief over Lazarus's death as he suffers with his friends. "Now when Mary came to where Jesus was and saw him, she fell at his feet, saying to him, 'Lord, if you had been here, my brother would not have died'" (John 11:32). Jesus responds not with remonstrance or rebuke but with tears. "When Jesus saw her weeping, and the Jews who had come with her also weeping, he was deeply moved in his spirit and greatly troubled. And he said, 'Where have you laid him?' They said to him, 'Lord, come and see.' Jesus wept. So the Jews said, 'See how he loved him!'" (11:33–36). Nothing of what he sees of their grief surprises him. He arrived in full knowledge that Lazarus was dead and that in short order he would Lazarus from the dead. Yet, despite his transcendent knowledge of God's power and purposes at work in the situation, he suffers with them.

The most shocking idea in the Christian religion, an idea foreign to all other systems of belief, is that the utterly transcendent God, who exists outside time, all-powerful and all-knowing, the self-existent one who needs nothing from anyone or anything, should condescend to be in our midst as one of us. In Jesus, God becomes man. It is almost unimaginable that such a God, high and lifted up, should dwell with us, should be concerned for us, should know us, and should care for us. It feels like the ultimate too-good-to-be-true fairytale story, a kind of wishful thinking on steroids. Conscious as we are of our limits, our imperfections, our frailty, we are naturally inclined to believe that God is interested in us only in proportion to what we have to offer him. The thought that he still cares for us when we have nothing to offer is simply unbelievable.

Suffering brings us the possibility of seeing the true depths of God's love for us. Suffering arises as illness puts limits on our abilities and on our lives. We feel our loss, and we feel increasingly useless. That God would be present with us in our pain, that he would enter into our pain, that he would suffer with us (literally, that we would see his com-passion), reveals just how much we are loved by God. And because love is value in action, through that unspeakable love we discover the true depths of our own value and worth in his sight.

Jesus's response to suffering brings us what we truly need. We do not really need freedom from suffering. We need love. We yearn to enjoy others and to be enjoyed, we yearn to know others and to be known by them, we yearn to flourish in community as part of community and to be valued by the community and to see our value through the community's valuing of us. We cannot flourish alone. Suffering and illness can lead us to despair of enjoying those good things; they threaten our ability to participate in the community, and they threaten our value to our community. Too easily we value ourselves in terms of our usefulness to our community. Suffering and illness threaten us with uselessness and therefore with worthlessness. But suffering also opens up new possibilities for loving and being loved that were not otherwise available to us. In our suffering, we may experience and know that God loves us, not because of our usefulness (our extrinsic value) but because of just how valuable we really are (our intrinsic value). Suffering forces us to cast ourselves on the one who gave us for himself, and in him we find all that we truly need: overflowing love, rest, and satisfaction for our weary souls.

Escape from Despair

Augustine famously prayed, "You have made us for Yourself, and our hearts find no peace until they rest in you."[32] We were made to know and be with God, to enter into the happy community of Father, Son, and Holy Spirit. Suffering cannot rob us of this purpose. Suffering cannot rob us of the pleasure and privilege of knowing and being with God. In our suffering we see more clearly that there is nothing better than to be with God, and him to be with us. Those who know this God and are known by him have escaped despair. We do not need a doctor to grant us a timely death to conquer suffering, for our suffering has been conquered by true life.

VI

Entrusting Ourselves to a Faithful Creator

P HYSICIAN-ASSISTED DEATH IS a profoundly weighty matter, for it raises timeless questions about the meaning and value of our lives, the problem of suffering, and the possibility and nature of human existence beyond the grave. At bottom, the question of assisted death is a question about the nature of human value and how we are to dignify that value in ourselves and in others. Those who by virtue of their professional commitments as doctors accept responsibility for the suffering of others feel a weighty responsibility to "do something." Faced with incurable suffering, we feel the temptation to take matters into our own hands, as it were, "to take arms against a sea of troubles, and by opposing end them."

In this book, I have offered a series of arguments against physician-assisted death. This presentation is not intended to be a comprehensive case against the practice; we have not considered the specific question of a doctor's professional ethic, as to whether deliberately acting to cause death can be reconciled with one's commitment to profess healing. Nor have we considered the various slippery-slope arguments against assisted death, arguments that cite concerns over the potential exploitation and vulnerability of marginalized populations, or the inevitable and natural expansion of the practice when causing death comes to be regarded as an accepted and effective form of medical intervention for untreatable physical and mental illness. These arguments are very important, but I have focused on the primary question of whether it is ever, under any circumstances, appropriate to cause death in order to relieve suffering. If causing death could, in principle, be a good thing to do under certain conditions, then concerns about slippery slopes seem to be comparatively weaker grounds for opposing the relief of suffering through assisted death. I have aimed to go straight to the heart of the matter: to show that causing death to relieve suffering cannot be justified in principle under any conditions.

The arguments presented in this book can be summarized in the following theses.

Theses

1. Because physician-assisted death intentionally aims to cause the death of the patient, it is distinctly different from other practices in end-of-life medical care.

2. Patients seek physician-assisted death because life with suffering seems pointless to them.

3. People have intrinsic value, not merely extrinsic value.

4. If people have intrinsic value, it is not appropriate to intentionally end their existence.

5. Physician-assisted death devalues people.

6. Value based on personal autonomy can only be extrinsic and conditional value.

7. In using death as a remedy for suffering, physician-assisted death presumes to know what it is like to be dead.

8. The arguments for physician-assisted death presuppose truths about human nature and ultimate reality that undercut those same arguments.

9. To live with suffering, we need transcendent meaning rather than self-invented meaning.

10. We know by nature that we matter, but we only clearly behold the true meaning and significance of our lives in the life, death, resurrection, and ascension of Christ.

The Theses Defended

1. Because physician-assisted death intentionally aims to cause the death of the patient, it is distinctly different from other practices in end-of-life medical care.

Physician-assisted death refers to intentional and deliberate actions on the part of the physician aimed at causing the death of the patient. This intentional aiming at death clearly distinguishes physician-assisted death from other practices in end-of-life medical care such as palliative care, terminal sedation, or withholding or withdrawing life-sustaining therapies.

The specific moral question we are addressing is whether it is permissible and justifiable to deliberately cause the death of a patient when the patient has voluntarily requested the doctor to do so. The doctor may cause the patient's death directly by administering a lethal dose of drug intravenously, or indirectly by providing the patient with a prescription for a lethal dose of drug that the patient ingests on their own. In both cases, the physician is acting in order to cause death. Death is the express goal of the physician's action. This intentionality is the defining feature of physician-assisted death. Physician-assisted death is therefore closely akin to suicide, even if the process involves external input and an external agent.

In criticizing the practice of physician-assisted death, I do not intend to suggest that these other practices are unethical. Indeed, they are often profoundly ethical provided they are performed in the right manner, at the right time, and for the right reasons. One of the important tasks of the physician is to judge when and how to care for patients by intervening less aggressively, rather than more aggressively, and to determine what treatments are helpful or unhelpful to those who are dying. Palliative medicine, the legacy of a Christian physician named Dame Cicely Saunders, has proven effective at helping seriously ill patients enjoy life to the fullest possible extent as they journey toward death.

2. *Patients seek physician-assisted death because life with suffering seems pointless to them.*

Patients seek physician-assisted death not primarily because of physical suffering or uncontrolled pain, but rather because life with suffering seems pointless to them in light of a loss of autonomy, independence, or sense of meaning and purpose.

Survey data presented in this book demonstrate that uncontrolled physical pain and symptoms are far from the main reasons that patients seek physician-assisted death. Rather, patients seek death because of concerns over loss of autonomy and independence, a fear of being a burden, and sense of meaningless and purposelessness in life. No less than other forms of suicide, a desire for physician-assisted death is an expression of despair. Because these forms of suffering represent existential, psychological, and spiritual phenomena, they are far more difficult for doctors to address. Indeed, they are more properly addressed through pastoral care. Physician-assisted death represents a desperate attempt by doctors to overcome the spiritual challenges presented by suffering and death.

This entails that those who lack the spiritual resources required to face suffering and death will be far more likely to seek physician-assisted death. Indeed, social-scientific data suggest that those who typically seek physician-assisted death in Canada are wealthy, white, and nonreligious. Although such persons are not typically regarded as vulnerable because of their socioeconomic status, such an assessment of vulnerability is rather superficial. It seems plausible that their nonreligious outlook on life makes them profoundly vulnerable to the desire for death. Given that spiritual concerns about the purpose of life in the face of suffering are determinative of the choice to seek physician-assisted death, an inability to sustain one's meaning and purpose in the face of suffering should count as the most important form of vulnerability to the desire for death.

3. People have intrinsic value, not merely extrinsic value.

We may distinguish between two basic forms of value, extrinsic and intrinsic value. Whereas we have extrinsic value by virtue of the things we can do, we have intrinsic value by virtue of what we are. Extrinsic value derives from utility; consequently, if that which has extrinsic value loses its utility, it also loses its value. That which has intrinsic value, by contrast, cannot lose its value, for its value derives simply from what it is. Intrinsic value is therefore unconditional value.

Things that have intrinsic value have two particular characteristics that help us to recognize that value: they are priceless and irreplaceable. For example, one might say that certain great works of art such as the *Mona Lisa* have intrinsic value. Given its historical, cultural, and artistic significance, you couldn't really put a price on such a work of art, and you certainly couldn't replace it if it were destroyed. The most pronounced example of these characteristics is, of course, people. People are priceless (any attempt to buy or sell them inevitably fails to recognize their worth; hence slavery is a great evil), and people are irreplaceable. We are each utterly unique in our person and in our value.

One important difference between intrinsic value and extrinsic value is that the former kind of value creates an obligation for us to manifest respect and appreciation for that value. In this sense, we say that intrinsic value is "value from inside," whereas extrinsic value is "value from outside. "Extrinsic value depends on our valuation of the object of value. Intrinsic value, on the other hand, commands our value and respect. If something is intrinsically valuable, we have no choice but to value it, and we are in the wrong if we fail to value it in accordance with its true value.

4. If people have intrinsic value, it is not appropriate to intentionally end their existence.

To understand the connection between intrinsic value and the wrongness of causing death, consider the following syllogism:

MAJOR	If something has intrinsic value, it is always good that it exists.
MINOR	If it is good for something to exist, it is not appropriate to end its existence.
CONCLUSION	Therefore, if people have intrinsic value, it is not appropriate to intentionally end their existence.

There is a deep connection between value and goodness of existence. To say that something has value is to say that it is good that it exists. This is easily appreciated by reversing the logic; if you say that it does not matter whether something exists, you are also saying that it is of no particular value. So we cannot value something without also valuing its existence.

Now, if something is intrinsically valuable, then its value is unconditional. And if its value is unconditional, then the value of its existence is unconditional. If something has intrinsic value, then it is unconditionally good that it exists.

So to suggest that it is better for something not to exist is necessarily to declare that it does not have intrinsic value. Claiming that it is good to end someone's existence implies that their existence is not unconditionally good; rather, the goodness of their existence is conditional. If this were the case, they could not possibly have intrinsic value.

But since we have established that people have intrinsic value, we are forced to conclude that their existence is unconditionally good. If this is the case, then it is never good for them to cease existing, and it is not appropriate to intentionally cause their death.

5. *Physician-assisted death devalues people.*

By endorsing a patient's desire for death, physician-assisted death affirms that it is not good for them to exist and denies that they have intrinsic value. Therefore, physician-assisted death devalues people.

This thesis is the simple corollary of the last. By declaring that it is in fact appropriate to cause the death of a particular kind of patient who meets prespecified eligibility criteria, physician-assisted death necessarily denies that it is unconditionally good for that person to exist. If the goodness of that person's existence is only conditional, then they do not have intrinsic value. And if the goodness of some people's existence is conditional on the desirability of their lives to them, then this is true for all of us. Hence the goodness of existence is conditional for all of us, and none of us have intrinsic value.

In this way, support for physician-assisted death forces us to deny that people have intrinsic value. It remains to us only to have extrinsic value, whether to ourselves or to anyone else. And since mere extrinsic value is a lesser and conditional form of value in comparison to intrinsic value, physician-assisted death detracts from human value. It devalues people.

6. Value based on personal autonomy can only be extrinsic and conditional value.

Basing respect for life on respect for personal autonomy does not equate to respect for intrinsic human value. Value based on personal autonomy can only be extrinsic and conditional value.

Founding the value of life on the obligation to respect personal autonomy entails that the goodness of a person's existence is conditional on their own personal satisfaction with life. While this may feel like a form of intrinsic value, since the valuation is independent of our own personal judgment, it is in fact a form of extrinsic value because the person's value is conditional on their own valuation. In this sense, founding respect for life on respect for autonomy invites people to regard themselves as means to their own ends. So long as their existence is useful to achieving their goals, it is of value. If their existence is no longer useful to them, then it is of no value. Therefore, offering to cause death out of respect for autonomy invites people to regard themselves as only conditionally valuable. Respect for autonomy does not equate to respect for intrinsic human value.

If we are priceless and irreplaceable, possessed of intrinsic value, then this is a fact that we must bear in mind of ourselves as well as of others. Indeed, it is the task of those who care for the sick and the suffering to remind them of the true depths of their value. We are to invite those who feel useless and weak and worthless to remember that they are priceless and irreplaceable. This is the highest motivation of medical care.

7. In using death as a remedy for suffering, physician-assisted death presumes to know what it is like to be dead.

Physician-assisted death purports to be an act of compassion or mercy. To claim that death is good for you, you have to make some assumption about what it is like to be dead. Uncertainty over what it is like to be dead famously prevented Hamlet from taking his own life in Shakespeare's play. Claiming to help someone by taking their life is boldly presumptuous. If and only if we know what it is like to be dead can we confidently assert that someone is better off dead.

The question is whether doctors have grounds for such knowledge of what it is like to be dead. In fact, this is a philosophical question, inaccessible to the empirical methods of medical science. Doctors cannot pronounce with any authority on whether there is life after death. Neither, indeed, can patients. Claims about the existence and nature of life after death will always be matters of speculation, apart from divine revelation, and this is just as true for those who deny the possibility of life after death as it is for those who believe in the possibility of life after death. Those who argue in favor of physician-assisted death do not typically cite Scripture or divine revelation in support of their position. Most advocates for the practice cite their atheistic commitments as motivation for their support for physician-assisted death.

Physician-assisted death should therefore be understood as an act of deep faith in one's personal philosophical convictions about the nature of ultimate reality and human existence. In this sense, it is very much a religious (if godless) practice, rather than a scientific, evidence-based practice.

8. The arguments for physician-assisted death presuppose truths about human nature and ultimate reality that undercut those same arguments.

Reason reflecting on nature compels us to conclude that humans are composed of both a material substance, the body, and an immaterial substance, the soul. Because the death of our material substance (the body) does not necessarily entail the death of our immaterial substance (the soul), it is entirely plausible that human existence and consciousness continue beyond physical death. Since apart from divine revelation we do not know what this existence is like, we are never justified in claiming on our own authority that someone is better off dead or that we are helping them by causing their death.

Except for the most recalcitrant and committed skeptics, very few express doubt as to the existence of the human body. By contrast, many would express real doubt that humans also have an immaterial soul. To them, the idea of the soul seems like a relic of the premodern, prescientific cultural past. This understanding of what we humans fundamentally are (body and soul, or body alone) is important to discussions about physician-assisted death, since those who believe that we are purely physical (we are bodies without souls) are naturally inclined to believe that once bodily function has ceased, further existence or consciousness is impossible. On the other hand, if we have a soul, and if this soul is conscious, then it seems distinctly plausible that there could be life beyond the death of our bodies.

In entertaining these questions, we are transported into the abstruse world of the philosophy of mind. Yet, as it turns out, the arguments are relatively straightforward. If we were merely physical bodies, we would have to deny the possibility that our thought processes function according to reason and logic. If thought processes are only physical neurons

firing electrical discharges, they would be entirely determined by the laws of physics and chemistry; we would have
no real choice as to what to think. For the same reason, we
would have no free will to decide what to do or to choose
freely; we would be mere robots behaving according to pre-
defined algorithms wired in our brains.

The problem, of course, is that we really do think, and
we trust our thinking. We really do make free choices, and
we hold others responsible for the choices they make. So we
can't just be physical objects. The only alternative is that we
have a real mind, an immaterial substance that is the basis
for our thinking and willing.

One example of such thinking and willing is deciding to
request physician-assisted death. Those who support physician-assisted death claim that the patient has, through
a thought process involving careful rational deliberation,
decided they are better off dead. And they are happy to
support this decision provided it is made freely and autonomously by the patient. But such claims are impossible if
we are merely physical objects. If we are merely physical
objects, we neither think nor freely will anything (autonomy would be a mere illusion). So, by its very nature, the
case for physician-assisted death presumes that we are both
body and soul. Since the existence of the soul would give
us a reason to doubt whether we are better off dead, we
can't support physician-assisted death without also having

a reason to oppose physician-assisted death. In this way, the practice is self-refuting.

9. To live with suffering, we need transcendent meaning rather than self-invented meaning.

The fundamental challenge of suffering is to sustain meaning and purpose in life. To that end, we need transcendent meaning rather than self-invented meaning.

When forced to journey through a valley of sorrow and suffering in life, we quickly find ourselves wondering whether there is any point to trudging on. When life is easy, pleasant, and pleasurable, it's easy to feel that it is good and worthwhile to be alive. Suffering challenges our sense of meaning and purpose in life. It forces us to come to terms with the reality that the meanings and purposes we invent for ourselves in life, whether through work or other pursuits, are more fiction than fact. If that meaning and that purpose are no longer within our grasp, we are brought face to face with the question of whether our existence has any real meaning or purpose that transcends our personal goals or desires. If our existence has a point that transcends our own personal projects, if we are part of a larger story, then we may find the strength to press on despite our sorrows. As Viktor Frankl puts it, "He who has a why to live can bear almost any how." But if our existence is merely much ado about nothing, then suffering forces us to confront the simple fact that life is useless and so are we.

Alasdair Macintyre observes, "Man is in his actions and practice, as well as in his fictions, essentially a story-telling animal." To make sense of our suffering and to bear up in the face of suffering, there needs to be a story behind and above our lives and our suffering. Macintyre continues, "The key question for men is not about their own authorship; I can only answer the question 'What am I to do?' if I can answer the prior question 'Of what story or stories do I find myself a part?'"[33] This is no less true when we confront the question, "Should I ask my doctor to end my life?" The answer depends on the story we find ourselves in and whether there is any story at all.

10. We know by nature that we matter, but we only clearly behold the true meaning and significance of our lives in the life, death, resurrection, and ascension of Christ.

Through reason reflecting on nature, we may dimly glimpse the truth that we are of profound value and that we exist for a purpose that transcends our personal desires and goals. But we only clearly behold the true meaning and significance of our lives in the life, death, resurrection, and ascension of Christ. Strengthened through the faith, hope, and love found in knowing Christ, we learn to see that our momentary life with suffering is not pointless but rather profoundly worthwhile.

Although it may be popular to insist that the only story for us is the story we write for ourselves, it's hard to deny that there must be some grand story of which we are a part. The mere fact that the cosmos exists strongly suggests that there must be some story. For why is it here if there is no story? Where could it possibly have come from? What made the Big Bang go bang? Moreover, that we have intrinsic value and that it is unconditionally good that we exist could only be true if we had some significant role in a story beyond ourselves. The existence of space and time, the intrinsic moral value of humans, and the glory and beauty of nature, with its intricate biological design and cosmic fine-tuning, bespeaks the presence of an Author of the universe. There is some story being written. We must have transcendent meaning, if only we would open our eyes to see it.

Christians are those who have discovered that Christ reveals the true logic behind all things. The story of Christ's life, death, resurrection, and ascension to glory makes sense of our momentary life with suffering. For our story is ultimately part of his story. Through faith in Christ, we are reconciled to God, and Christ's story becomes our own. Thus we find meaning, purpose, significance, and hope that transcends our circumstances and our pain. Faith in Christ gives us confidence that by his power and purposes he will vindicate our suffering. Hope in Christ gives us grace to patiently endure with eyes set on the eternal glory that we will soon enjoy with him. And the love of Christ satisfies our souls, for even better than a life free from suffering is a life lived in ever-deepening communion with God in Christ through the Holy Spirit. Soon our pilgrimage through this vale of tears will be ended, and our bodies will return to dust as we await God's new creation. Our only hope in life and death is that we belong, both body and soul, both in life and death, to our faithful Savior Jesus Christ. And until the Author of life brings our story on this earth to a close, we are wholeheartedly willing and ready to live for him.[34]

Therefore let those who suffer
according to God's will
entrust their souls to
a faithful Creator
while doing good.

1 Peter 4:19

Bibliography

Augustine. *Augustine: The City of God against the Pagans.* Cambridge Texts in the History of Political Thought. Cambridge: Cambridge University Press, 2021.

Augustine. *Confessions.* Translated by R.S. Pine-Coffin. London: Penguin Books, 1961.

Bennett, Gillian. "Goodbye & Good Luck!" August 18, 2014. https://deadatnoon.com.

Camus, Albert. *The Myth of Sisyphus.* Libros, 2015.

Chochinov, H. M., et al. "Dignity in the Terminally Ill: Revisited." *Journal of Palliative Medicine* 9, no. 3 (June 2006): 666–72.

Dees, M. K., Vernooij-Dassen, M. J., Dekkers, W. J., Vissers, K. C. & Weel, C. van. "'Unbearable suffering': a qualitative study on the perspectives of patients who request assistance in dying." *J Med Ethics* 37, 727 (2011).

Downar, J., et al. "Early experience with medical assistance in dying in Ontario, Canada: a cohort study." *CMAJ* 192, E173–E181 (2020).

Emanuel, E. J., Onwuteaka-Philipsen, B. D., Urwin, J. W. & Cohen, J. "Attitudes and Practices of Euthanasia and Physician-Assisted Suicide in the United States, Canada, and Europe." *JAMA* 316, 79–90 (2016).

Frankl, Viktor. *Man's Search for Meaning*. Boston: Beacon, 2006.

Groothuis, D. *Christian Apologetics: A Comprehensive Case for Biblical Faith*. Downers Grove, IL: InterVarsity Press, 2022.

Keller, Timothy. *Making Sense of God*. New York: Penguin, 2018.

Kilner, John F. "Special Connection and Intended Reflection." Pages 135-160 in *Why People Matter: A Christian Engagement with Rival Views of Human Significance*. Grand Rapids: Baker Academic, 2017.

Li, M. et al. "Medical Assistance in Dying—Implementing a Hospital-Based Program in Canada". *New England Journal of Medicine* 376 (2017): 2082–88.

Loggers, E. T. et al. "Implementing a Death with Dignity program at a comprehensive cancer center." *New England Journal of Medicine* 368 (2013): 1417–24.

MacIntyre, Alasdair. *After Virtue*. Notre Dame, IN: University of Notre Dame Press, 1981.

Meyer, Stephen. *Return of the God Hypothesis: Three Scientific Discoveries That Reveal the Mind behind the Universe*. San Francisco: HarperOne, 2021.

Nietzsche, Friedrich. *Thus Spake Zarathustra*. New York: Modern Library, 1917.

Perry, Tim. *Funerals: For the Care of Souls*. Bellingham, WA: Lexham Press, 2021.

Rosenberg, Alex. *The Atheist's Guide to Reality: Enjoying Life without Illusions*. New York: Norton, 2011.

Rubin, E. B., A. E. Buehler, and S. D. Halpern. "States Worse than Death among Hospitalized Patients with Serious Illnesses." *JAMA Internal Medicine* 176, no. 10 (2016): 1557–59.

Russell, B. *A Free Man's Worship*. Pages 70–76 in *The Basic Writings of Bertrand Russell*. London: Routledge, 2009.

Speed, D., et al. "What Do You Mean, 'What Does It All Mean?' Atheism, Non-religion, and the Meaning of Life." *SAGE Open* 8, no. 1 (2018). https://journals.sagepub.com/doi/10.1177/2158244017754238.

Sydenham, T. "Medical Observations Concerning the History and the Cure of Acute Diseases." In *The Works of Thomas Sydenham, M.D.* Translated by RG Latham. Sydenham Society, London. 1848. Available at https://medlib.bsmu.edu.ua/wp-content/uploads/2019/05/32.pdf.

Tolstoy, Leo. *My Confession*. London: Walter Scott, 1889.

NOTES

1. Invocation taken from Tim Perry, *Funerals: For the Care of Souls* (Bellingham, WA: Lexham Press, 2021), xix–xx.

2. See the statement by the American Association of Sociology, "Suicide is not the same as Physician Aid in Dying," available at https://ohiooptions.org/wp-content/uploads/2016/02/AAS-PAD-Statement-Approved-10.30.17-ed-10-30-17.pdfApproved-10.30.17-ed-10-30-17.pdf. Of note, AAS has now taken down this statement, see their more recent statement at https://suicidology.org/2023/03/08/aas-update-on-previous-statement/.

3. Li et al., NEJM 2017, Loggers et al. NEJM 2013.

4. Li et al. "Medical Assistance in Dying—Implementing a Hospital-Based Program in Canada." *New England Journal of Medicine* 376, 2082–88 (2017).

5. Dees et al. J Med Ethics 2011, Emanuel et al. JAMA 2016.

6. Emanuel et al. JAMA 2016, Downar et al. CMAJ 2020.

7. Gillian Bennett, "Goodbye & Good Luck!," August 18, 2014, https://deadatnoon.com.

8. https://www.commonlit.org/en/texts/no-man-is-an-island.

9. See John F. Kilner, "Special Connection and Intended Reflection," in *Why People Matter*, ed. John F. Kilner (Grand Rapids: Baker, 2017), 135–60.

10. Sydenham, *Medical Observations*, Preface to the first edition, page 25. Cited in this form in the preamble to

the constitution of the Christian Medical and Dental Association of Canada, https://cmdacanada.org/aboutcmda/.

11. Shakespeare, *Hamlet*, Act III, Scene I.

12. Shakespeare, *Hamlet*, Act III, Scene I.

13. K. Vonnegut, *The North American Review*, 267, no. 4 (Dec 1982): 46–49.

14. E. B. Rubin, A. E. Buehler, and S. D. Halpern, "States Worse than Death among Hospitalized Patients with Serious Illnesses," *JAMA Internal Medicine* 176, no. 10 (2016): 1557–59.

15. Alex Rosenberg, *The Atheist's Guide to the Universe* (New York: Norton, 2011), 236.

16. For futher discussion of the evidence for the resurrection of Jesus Christ from the dead, the interested reader may wish to read Groothuis, *Christian Apologetics*.

17. Frankl, *Man's Search for Meaning*, 76.

18. Camus, *The Myth of Sisyphus*, 6.

19. Frankl, *Man's Search for Meaning*, 76.

20. Frankl, *Man's Search for Meaning*, 75.

21. H. M. Chochinov et al., "Dignity in the Terminally Ill: Revisited," *Journal of Palliative Medicine* 9, no. 3 (June 2006): 666–72.

22. Timothy Keller, *Making Sense of God* (New York: Penguin, 2018), 65.

23. D. Speed et al., "What Do You Mean, 'What Does It All Mean?' Atheism, Non-religion, and the Meaning of Life," *SAGE Open* 8, no. 1 (2018), https://journals.sagepub.com/doi/10.1177/2158244017754238.

24. Leo Tolstoy, *My Confession*, 32.

25. Camus, *Myth of Sisyphus*, 7.

26. Keller, *Making Sense of God*, 64.

27. Shakespeare, *Macbeth,* Act V, Scene V.

28. Bertrand Russell, *A Free Man's Worship,* in *The Basic Writings of Bertrand Russell* (London: Routledge, 2009), 70–76.

29. Interested readers may wish to consult Stephen Meyer, *Return of the God Hypothesis: Three Scientific Discoveries That Reveal the Mind behind the Universe* (San Francisco: HarperOne, 2021).

30. For a detailed and accessible delineation of this argument, see Douglas Groothuis, chapter 18, "The Uniqueness of Humanity," in *Christian Apologetics,* 2nd ed. (Downers Grove, IL: InterVarsity Press, 2022).

31. Augustine, *The City of God against the Pagans,* 1182.

32. Augustine, *Confessions,* 21.

33. MacIntyre, *After Virtue,* 201.

34. Words from these last two sentences are drawn from the Heidelberg Catechism, question 1.